OWww!

TRAVELING WITH CHRONIC PAIN

WRITTEN & ILLUSTRATED BY

WENDY BROWN

Cover design by wendy brown

Book design by

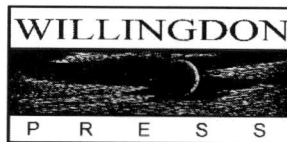

WILLINGDON
P   R   E   S   S

First Edition

ISBN-10: 1539388964
ISBN-13: 978-1539388968

DEDICATION

For Jocelyn Laurence

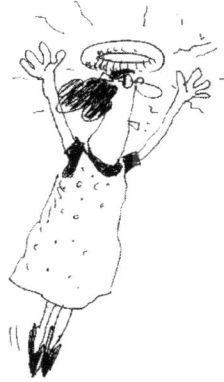

CONTENTS

ACKNOWLEDGMENTS

I would like to thank my sister, Shelley Brown, for suggesting the idea for this book, for being my first reader and critic, for her unflaggingly generous support and for being my best friend (and alternate Travel Saint).

I'd also like to thank Jocelyn Laurence for her tireless editing and for her companionship and understanding — not only as the (official) Travel Saint but as a sister-in-arms through hell and high tides. I will miss her forever.

Thanks as well to my friend and business partner, Janet Southcott, without whom this book would never have come to market.

And finally, thanks to my darling son Jack, my much-missed mother and father and all my excellent friends and relatives who put up with the vagaries of my chronic pain.

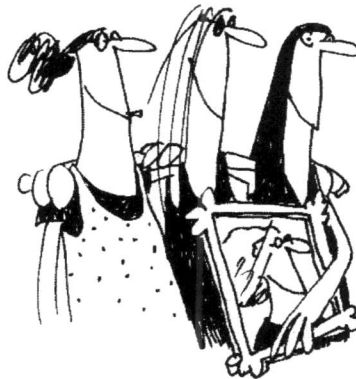

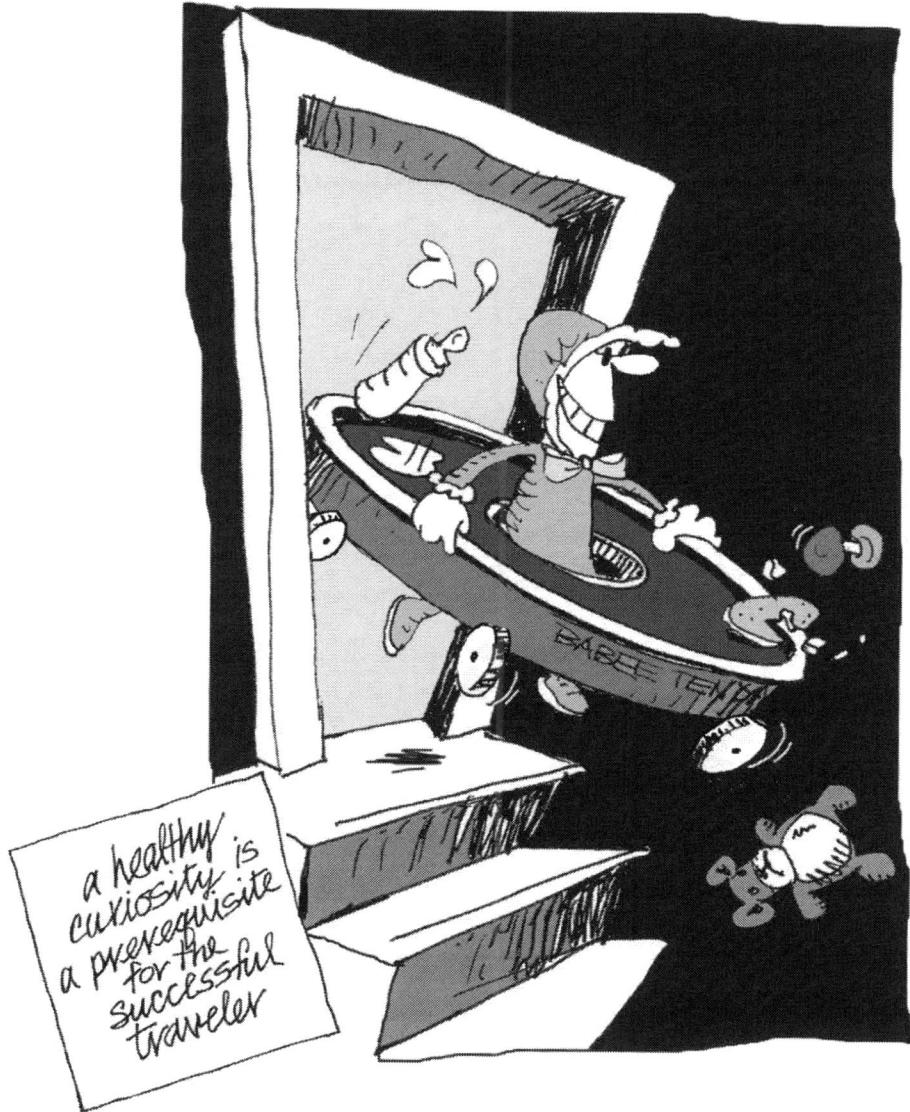

a healthy curiosity is a prerequisite for the successful traveler

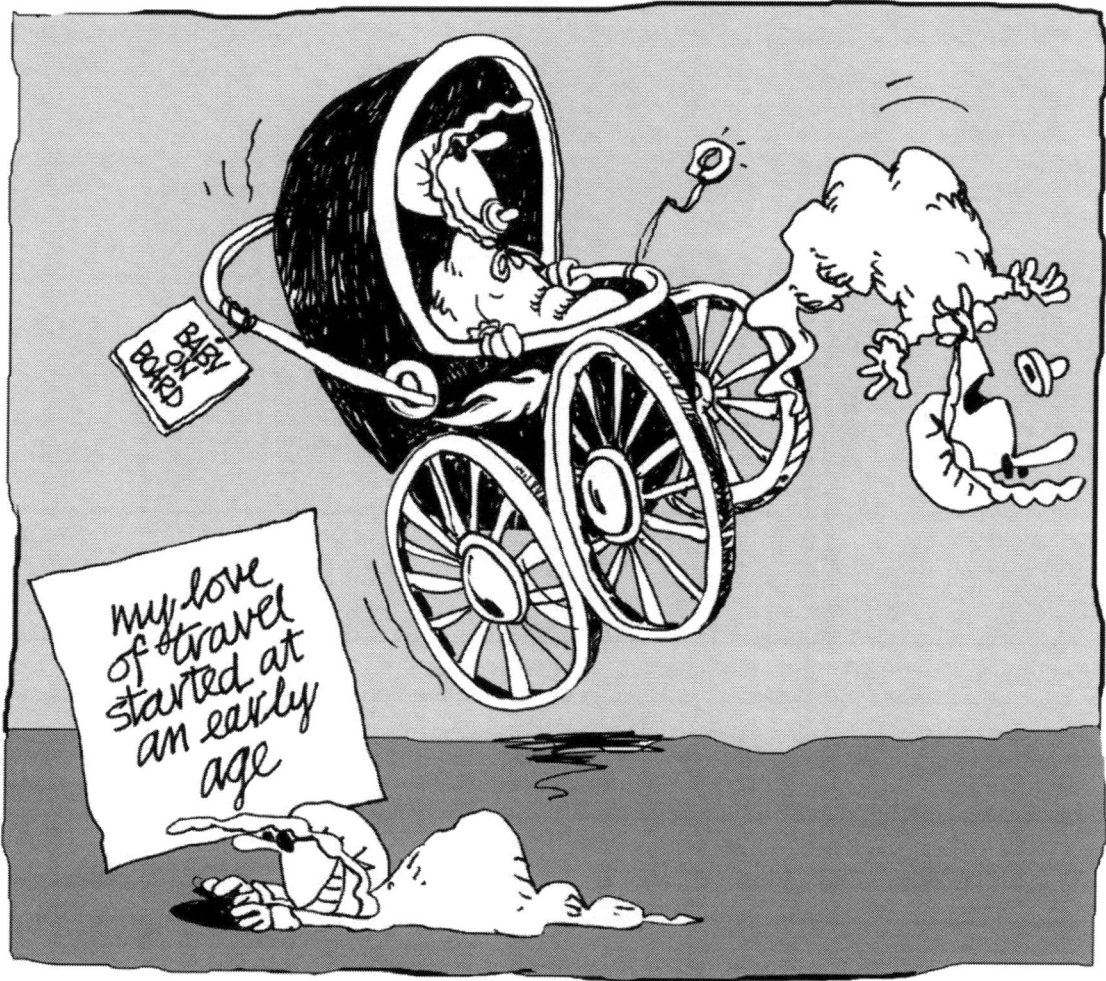

Or maybe my love of travel started at 18 when I rode 5,000 miles on the back of a motorcycle with my boyfriend—reading, painting my nails blue and sometimes sleeping—with a constant migraine. Not something I'd recommend now, but I was young and in love. And very dexterous. Or maybe it started when I was two and my parents ripped me away from my beloved Vancouver, moving me 3,000 miles by train across Canada to Ontario. Who knows? But neither chronic pain nor lack of funds has ever stopped me from traveling.

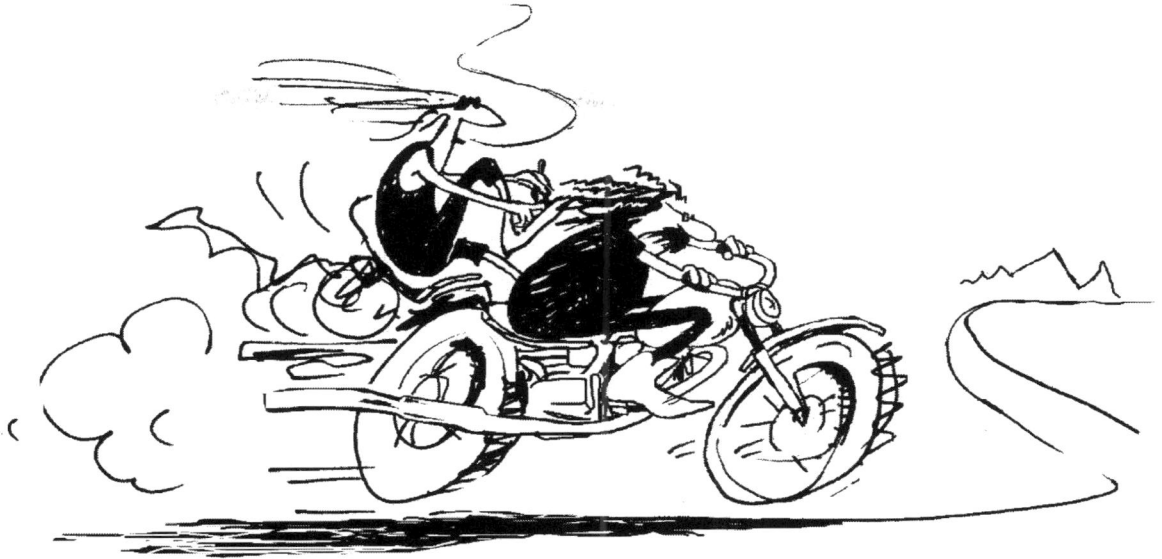

Although this book is about traveling with chronic pain, it's even more about empowerment. If you have chronic pain of any kind, you'll almost certainly have become your own expert in the subject. You'll have gone to endless doctors, read everything you can on the condition, tried all kinds of cures, both medical and alternative. Because chronic pain is devastating. It's limiting. It's ongoing. And if you've ever heard those seven crushing words from your specialist, "You'll just have to live with it," it's incredibly difficult to know *how* you're supposed to live with it.

Of course we always hope that someone will come up with a cure, but in the meantime we have to live around it.

My particular daily chronic pain is headache: migraines, cluster headaches, facial neuralgia and tension headaches. The pain makes it very difficult to lead a normal life. But I've always been a contrary type, and as a cartoonist, tend to see the humorous side to life. I also love to travel. So I've figured out ways to make life more or less work for me in spite of chronic pain—and I've figured out ways to travel that take into account the limitations caused by that pain.

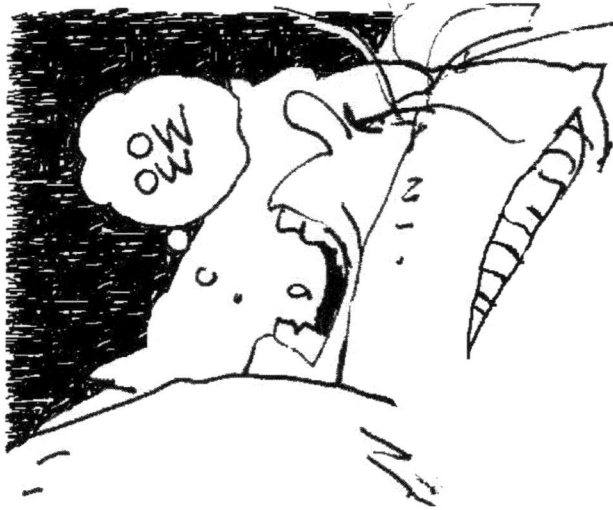

This book can't tell you how to live or travel with specific pain: arthritis, migraine, back or knee pain. The assumption is you know about your own condition and what works, what doesn't. It can't tell you specifically how to travel to Spain, Norway or the Antarctic. You will need to do your own research on the destination of your dreams. But it will help you believe that you can travel and what to do to minimize the limitations imposed by chronic pain.

What I basically want to say in this book is, "Yes you can!" Yes, you can travel with chronic pain. Yes, you can do things that other people do. Your life and travel will be affected by your condition, but it doesn't have to so limit you that you never leave home. It might require you to go about it a little differently, might require some forethought, but it absolutely is possible.

The trouble with having major pain every day is that it eventually makes us want to give up. Makes us want to just curl into ourselves, never take on anything that might exacerbate the pain. But giving in makes our life so dull, so boring and unfulfilling that we might as well not be alive at all. The dread depression sets in and we just don't want to go on.

It's not necessary to respond in this way. We can do things, can go places, can accomplish goals. Maybe not in exactly the same way as people without chronic pain, but by designing our lives to accommodate the pain, we can do almost anything other people take for granted.

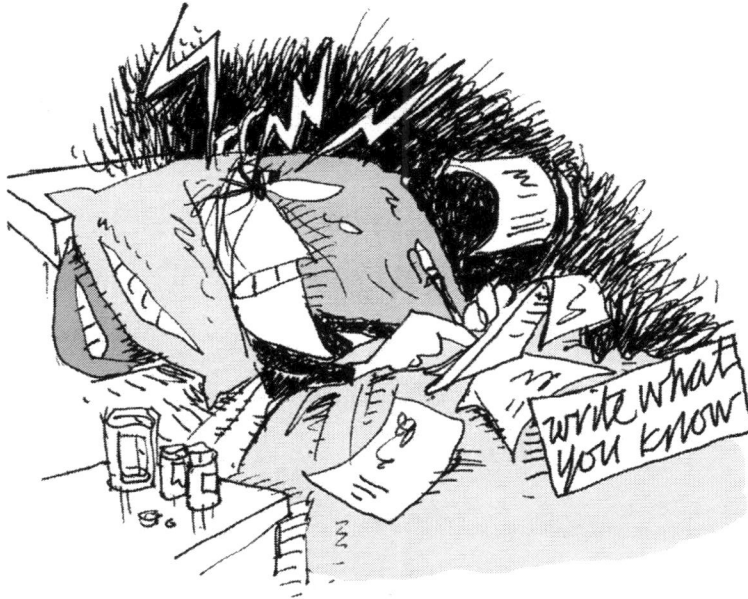

It's a pretty serious subject. But because I'm a cartoonist (and because they say a picture is worth a thousand words) I've done a lot of the book in cartoons. Laughter is good for almost any ailment, and I believe if we can keep our sense of humor—even about our own pain—we can live with it. And quite often rise above it.

People living with chronic pain are not usually considered disabled in the same way as people confined to a wheelchair or bed. Most of us don't have obvious mobility issues, don't generally carry any visible signs of our daily pain, but we are nevertheless disadvantaged. Chronic pain makes daily life difficult. And of course, it makes travel even more difficult. But with a few thoughtful concessions, not impossible.

The most important thing I've learned about traveling with chronic pain is not to overdo it. There's a tendency to push yourself way beyond your limit—you don't want to miss anything, right? But whether traveling alone or with a friend, the last thing you want is to end up in a foreign emergency ward begging for drugs:

You're going to waste far more time in flat-out agony than you would if you just took to your bed now and then, and

They almost certainly won't give you anything better than the drugs you already have with you—and might call the police, either because you're acting like a lunatic or they think you're a drug addict.

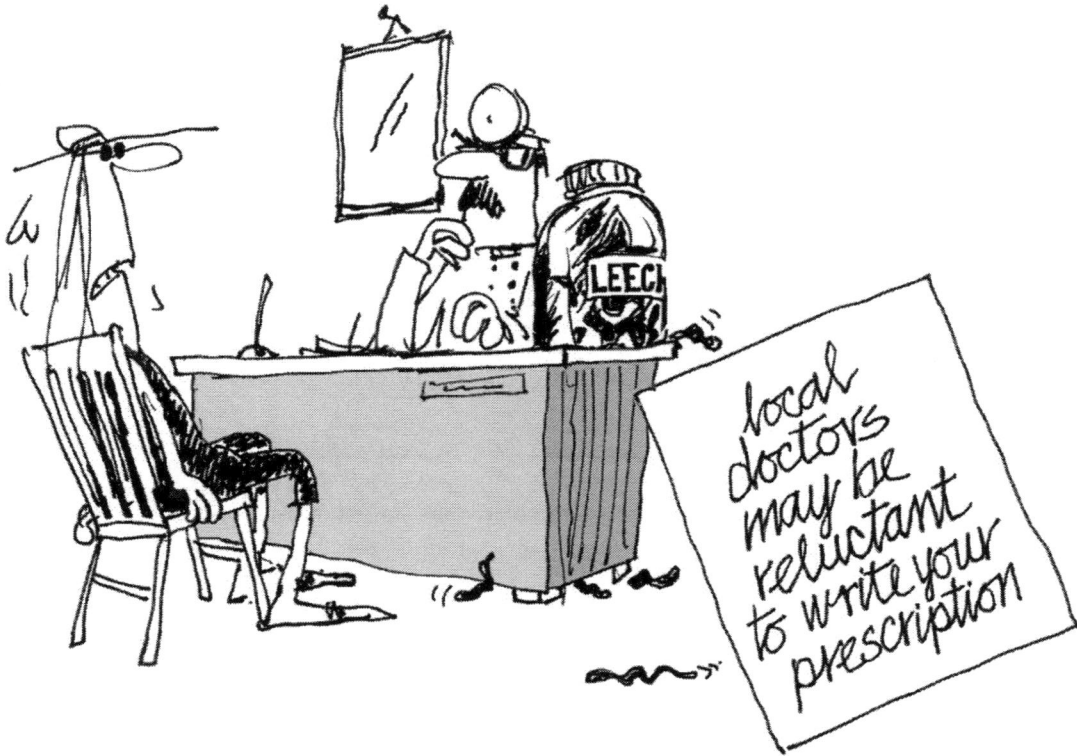

local doctors may be reluctant to write your prescription

Neither is good. So build in a little downtime, miss a monument or two while your friends go on without you, and have a fabulous holiday. Oh, and snap photos. If you take a lot of meds for your pain, you might not clearly remember everywhere you've been and your photos will be a happy reminder of the fun you've had.

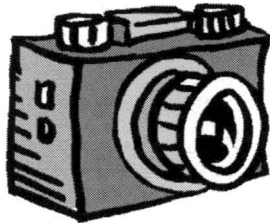

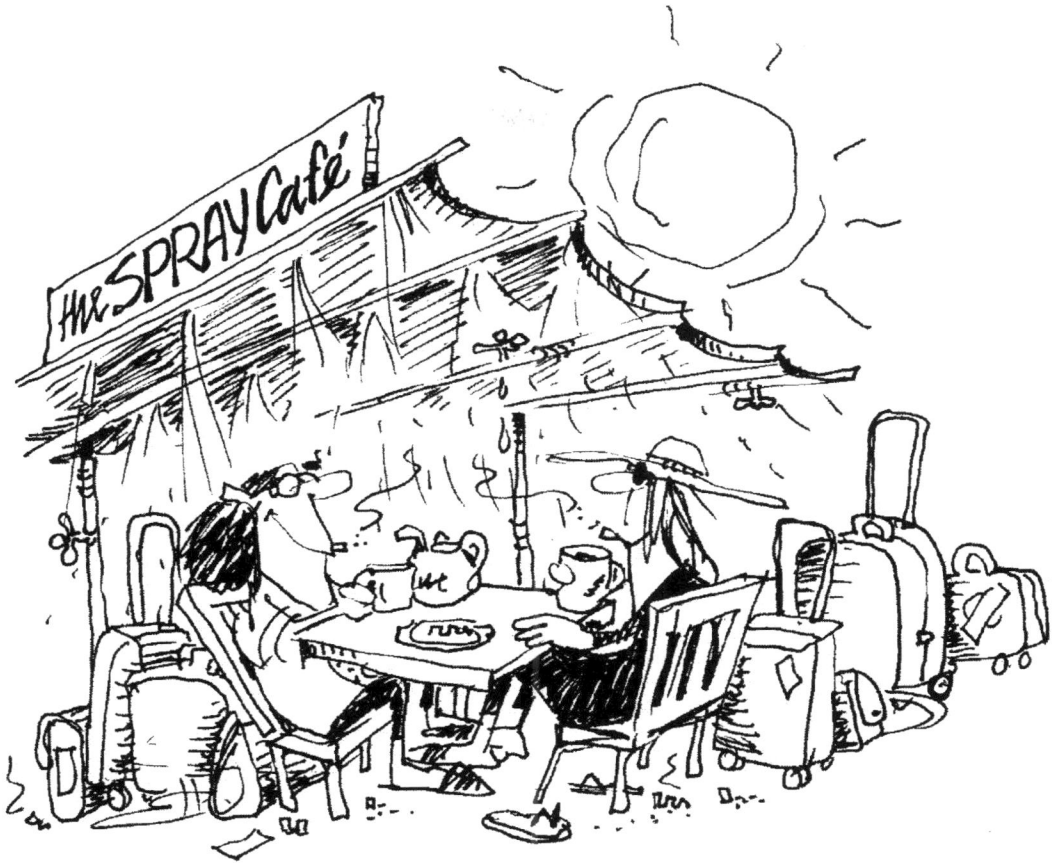

SEVILLE 2012

You might notice that my friend the Travel Saint and I are smoking everywhere in the cartoons. For years we both smoked constantly, and though it's become increasingly difficult to find decent smoking spots, we both continue to try. (Doctors used to prescribe nicotine for migraines. And caffeine. Maybe they knew something we no longer do. Of course, leeches haven't been a huge success . . .) I've recently taken up the electronic vapor cigarette in an attempt to quit, and I must admit, travel is significantly easier without the endless need to smoke.

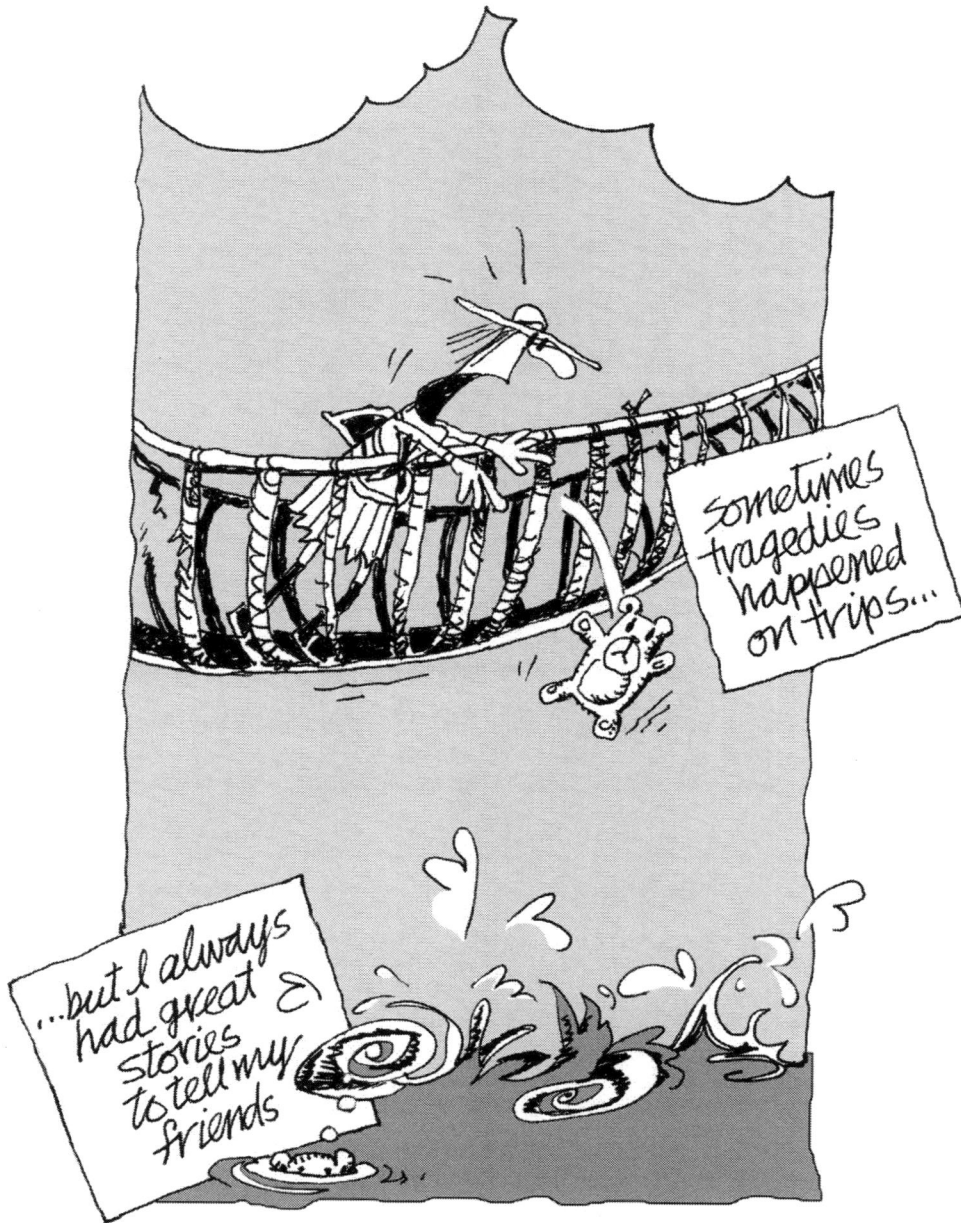

I hope my travel tips are of some use to you. And that you'll be inspired to pack up your meds, find your own Travel Saint and get out there into the big, bad, wonderful world in spite of your chronic pain. I figure if you're going to be in pain anyway, you might as well be in pain somewhere interesting.

OWww!

Good luck and happy trails to you!

wendy

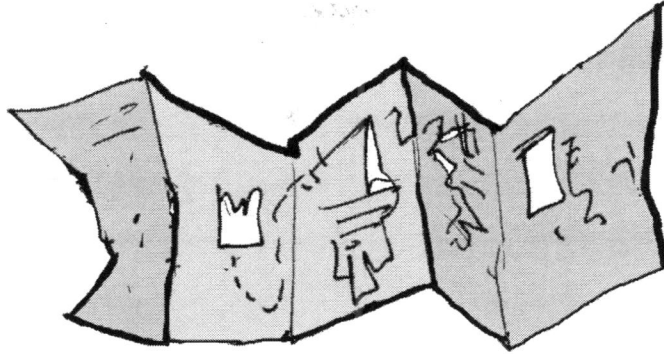

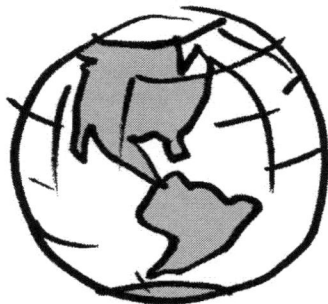

Chapter 1
WHERE TO GO

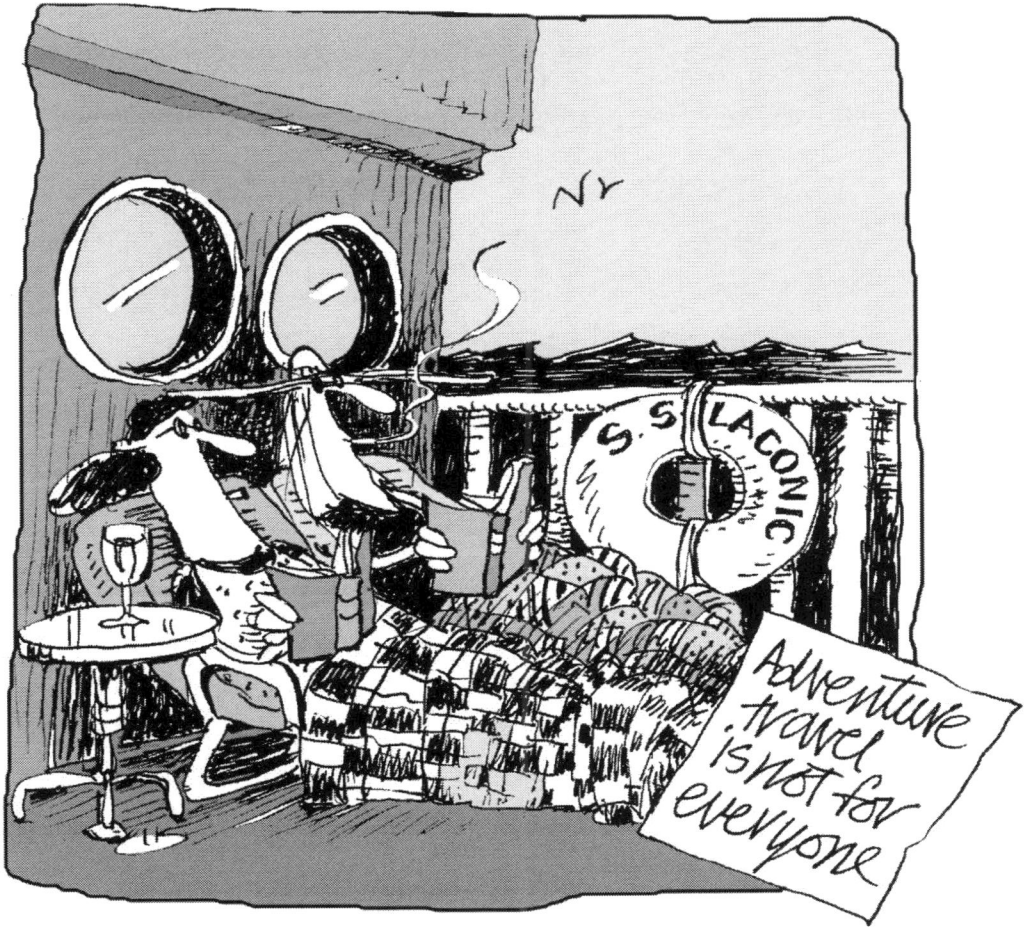

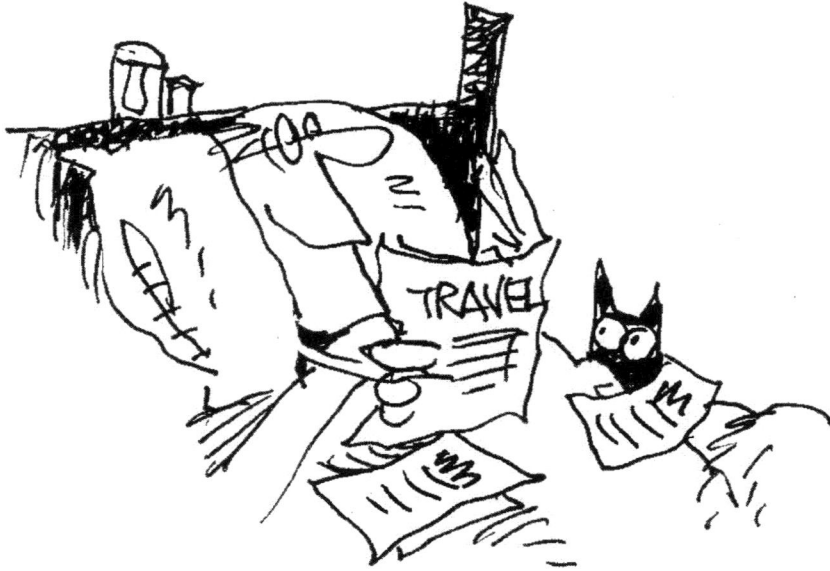

It's not so much where *you go as* how *you go*

Sometimes it feels like the closest we'll get to going anywhere is lying in bed, watching a travel show on TV. There are days when the pain is too great to even imagine being anywhere other than home. But other days, when the pain lessens somewhat and the longing to be somewhere exotic kicks in, pick up the phone and call a travel agent or go online and book somewhere fabulous. You CAN travel! Yes, there might be bad days when you're away. But there are bad days no matter where you are. As long as you pick a place that provides the services and comforts your pain management requires, you'll be fine!

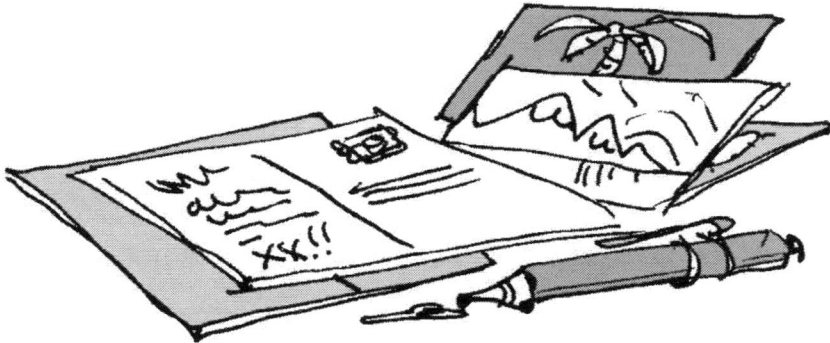

How to Choose Your Destination

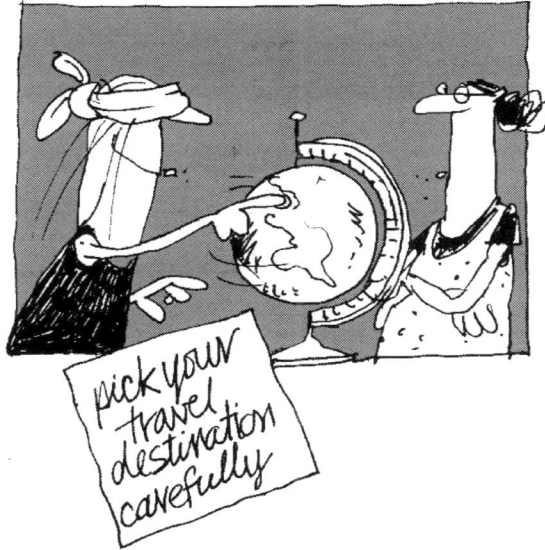

When chronic pain is a travel consideration, some locations are better than others. Generally speaking, it's best to avoid any destination or travel package that contains the word "adventure." This includes remote camping, river rafting, mountain climbing, physical extremes of any kind . . . and war zones.

Think about what you need:

You need to be as comfortable as possible so nothing external intensifies your normal pain level.

You need a decent bed to lie in when you're in too much pain to go out—not to mention getting a good night's sleep.

You may need a temperate climate or major air-conditioning.

You'll need available, ready-to-eat food for the times you're just not up to cooking or searching endlessly for a restaurant.

Some of us need quiet.

Some need professional massages.

You know what you require to keep you as active and pain-free as possible.

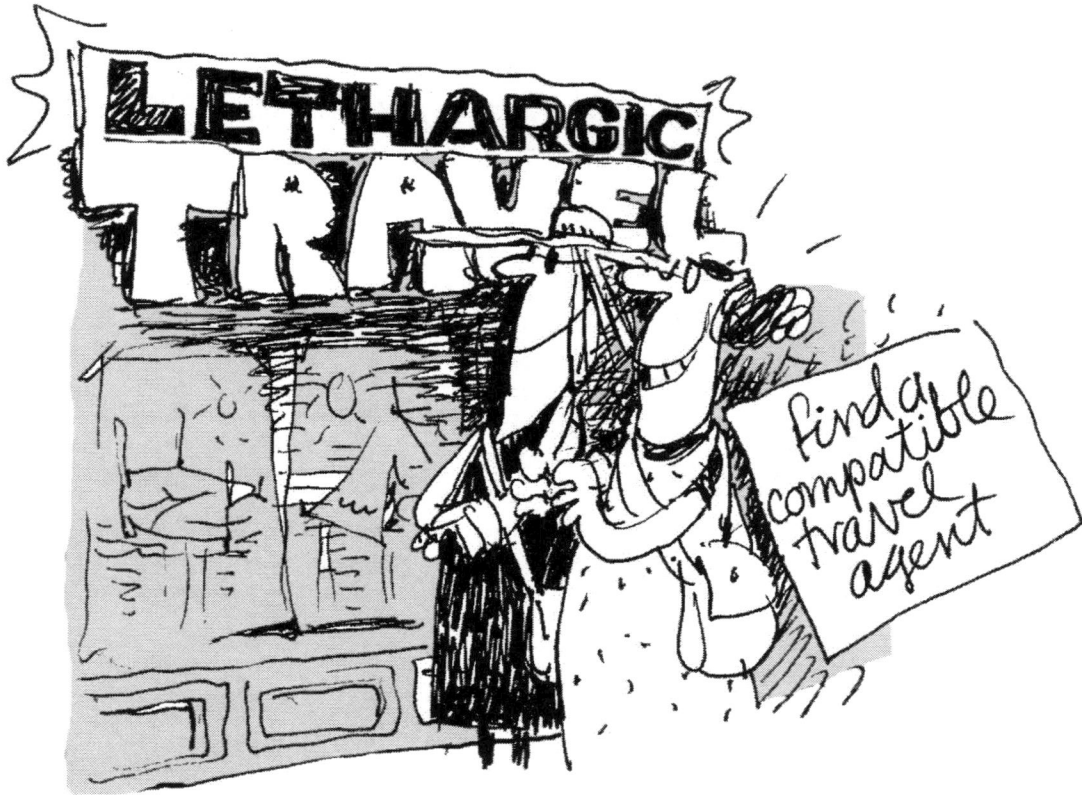

Be willing to compromise on some of the less important details—if you want absolutely everything to be the same as at home, you'd probably be better off staying there.

Some destinations are more favorable than others when chronic pain is a consideration. Places with serious temperature extremes are not always a good choice, although with central air, efficient heating and clothing designed for extreme weather, you have more choices than ever before.

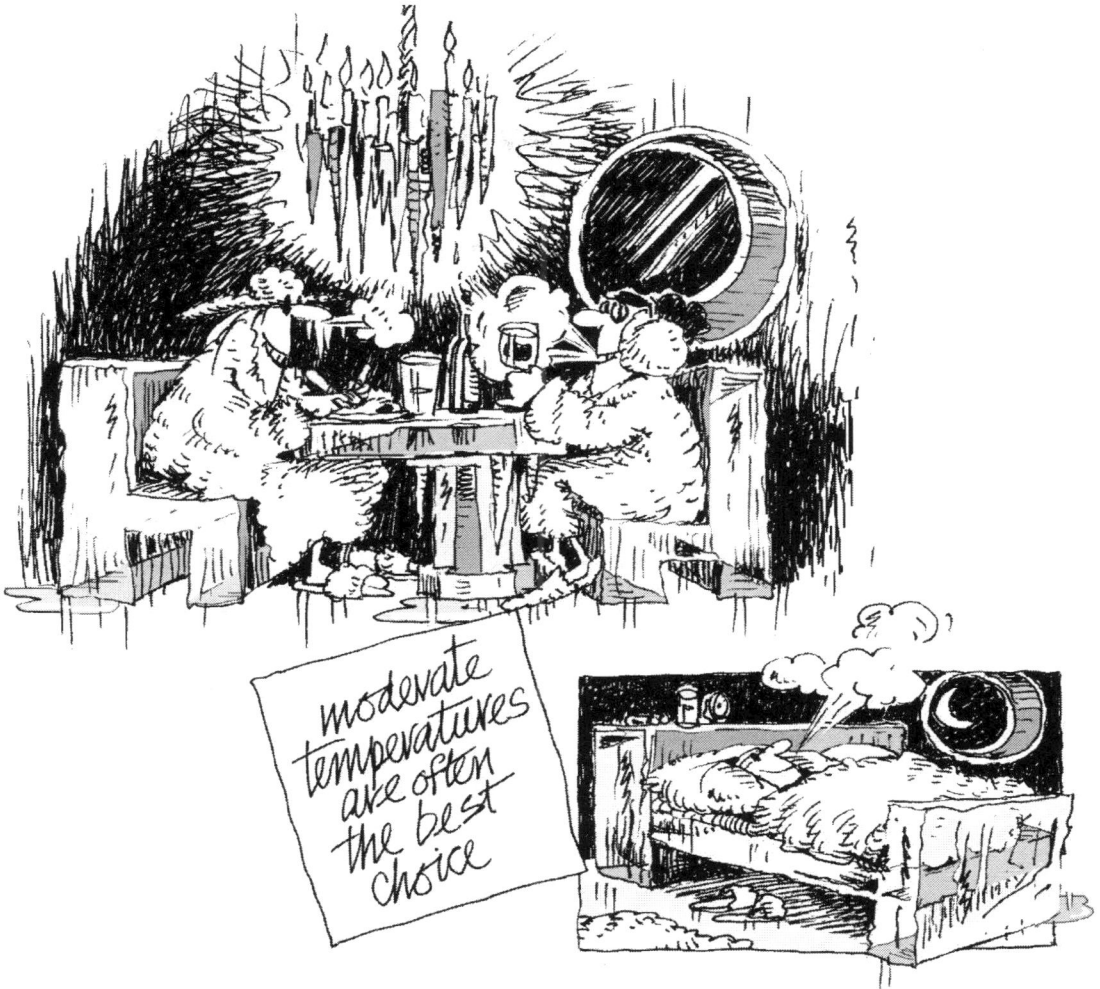

moderate temperatures are often the best choice

Remember, though, you have to go outside sometimes. As the Boy Scouts say, "Be Prepared."

Tours, which at first glance might seem ideal, often aren't. Cramming so many places into the itinerary, the average tour has to move along at quite a clip, often rousing you from your bed at some ungodly hour and hustling you onto a bus at first light. They don't like to wait while you wander around loosening the night kinks, taking your meds and gradually getting used to the pain of yet another day. Chances are, with your blessings, the tour will grind on without you, and you'll have paid all that money for nothing.

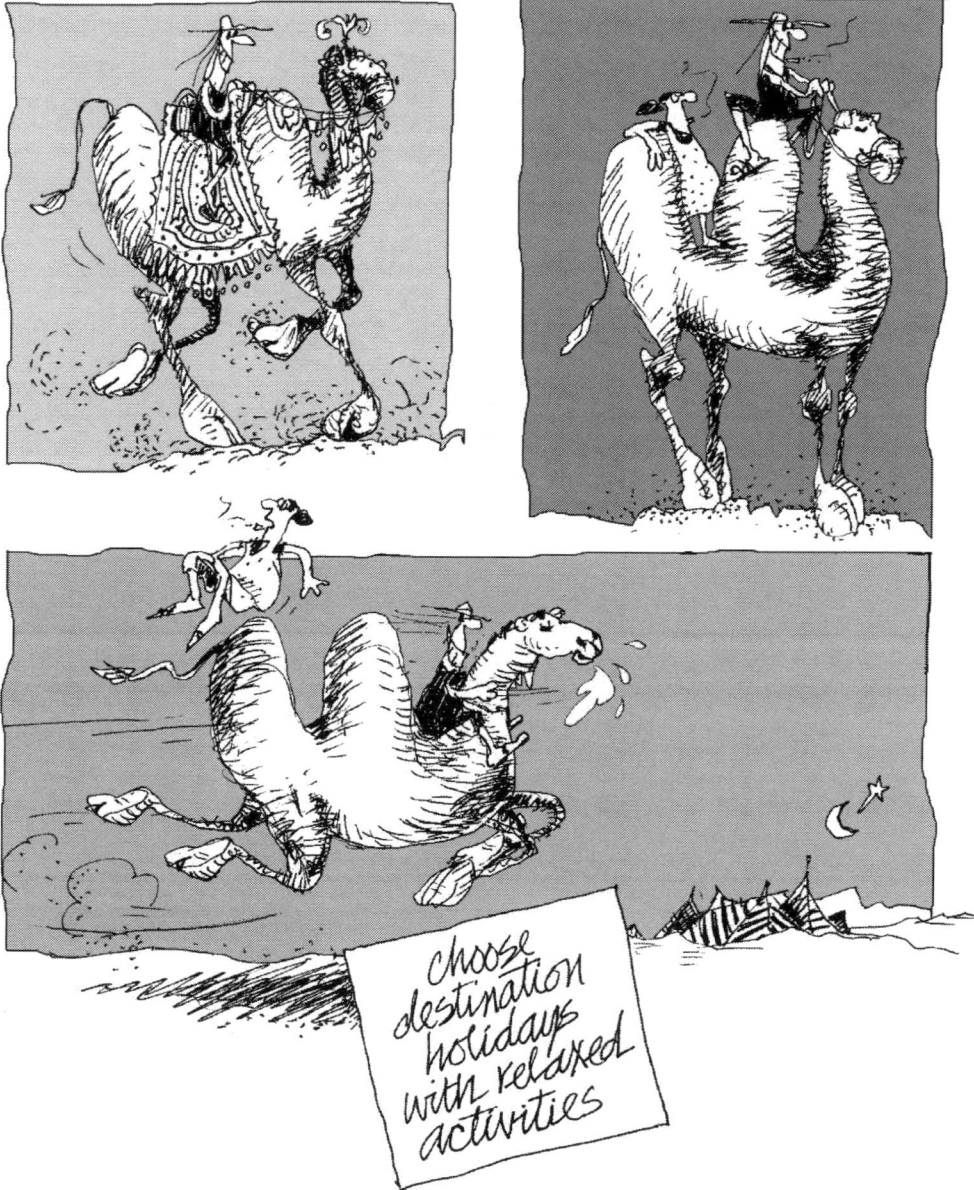

choose
destination
holidays
with relaxed
activities

Cruises are especially well suited to life with chronic pain. How bad can it be when your bedroom travels with you? Plentiful food is available at all hours, spas and entertainment are on board, not to mention the ship's doctor, and if you're not up to leaving the ship while in port, a new landfall will soon loom into sight.

Many different theme cruises are available (classic-movie lovers, senior singles, moon-rock enthusiasts) so you should be able to find one targeted to your specific interests. There may be only one real drawback to cruising. The big ships are the size of a small city, so if walking is painful, that could be a disadvantage, although the staff is usually very helpful. You can avoid the stairs on larger ships with elevators, and you can always arrange for a wheelchair.

Much like cruises, all-inclusive resorts attempt to cater to your every need. Most resorts also provide day trips so you can see some of the surrounding area if you wish. It's a stress-free introduction to a country and you can always return for a slightly less structured holiday if you fall in love with the place.

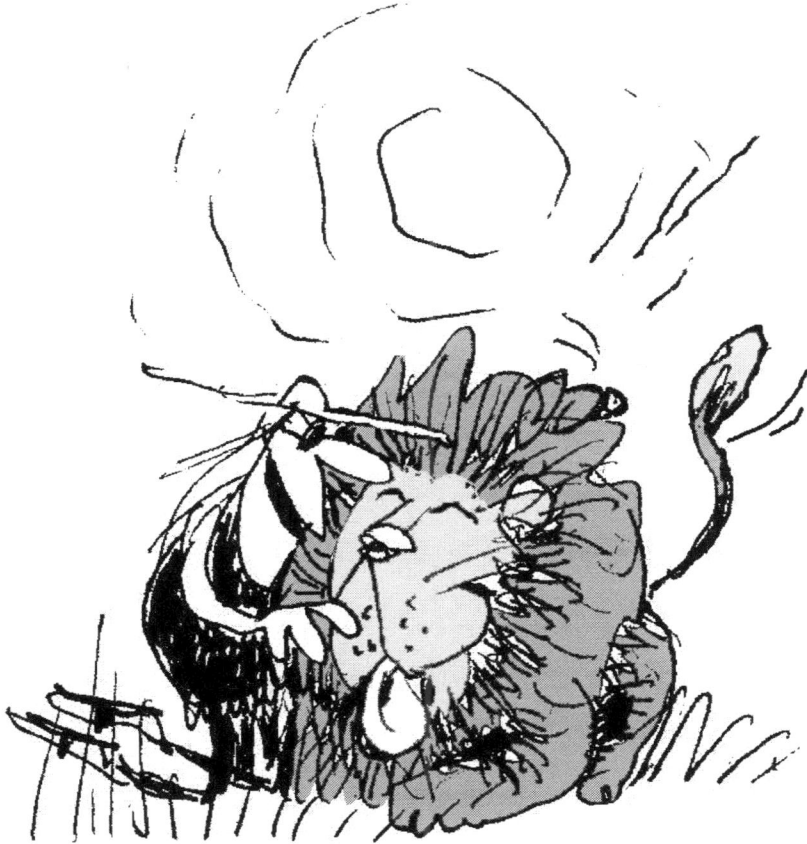

So many travel destinations are accessible to people with various disabilities that we can now travel almost everywhere. It's not so much where you go as how you go. Take your time, remember to plan for your comfort needs and be ready to put up with a little less ease now and then in return for a fabulous experience.

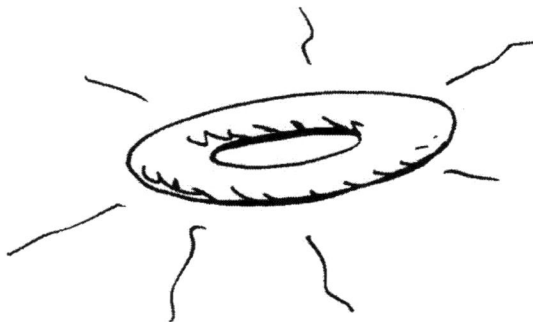

Chapter 2
THE TRAVEL SAINT

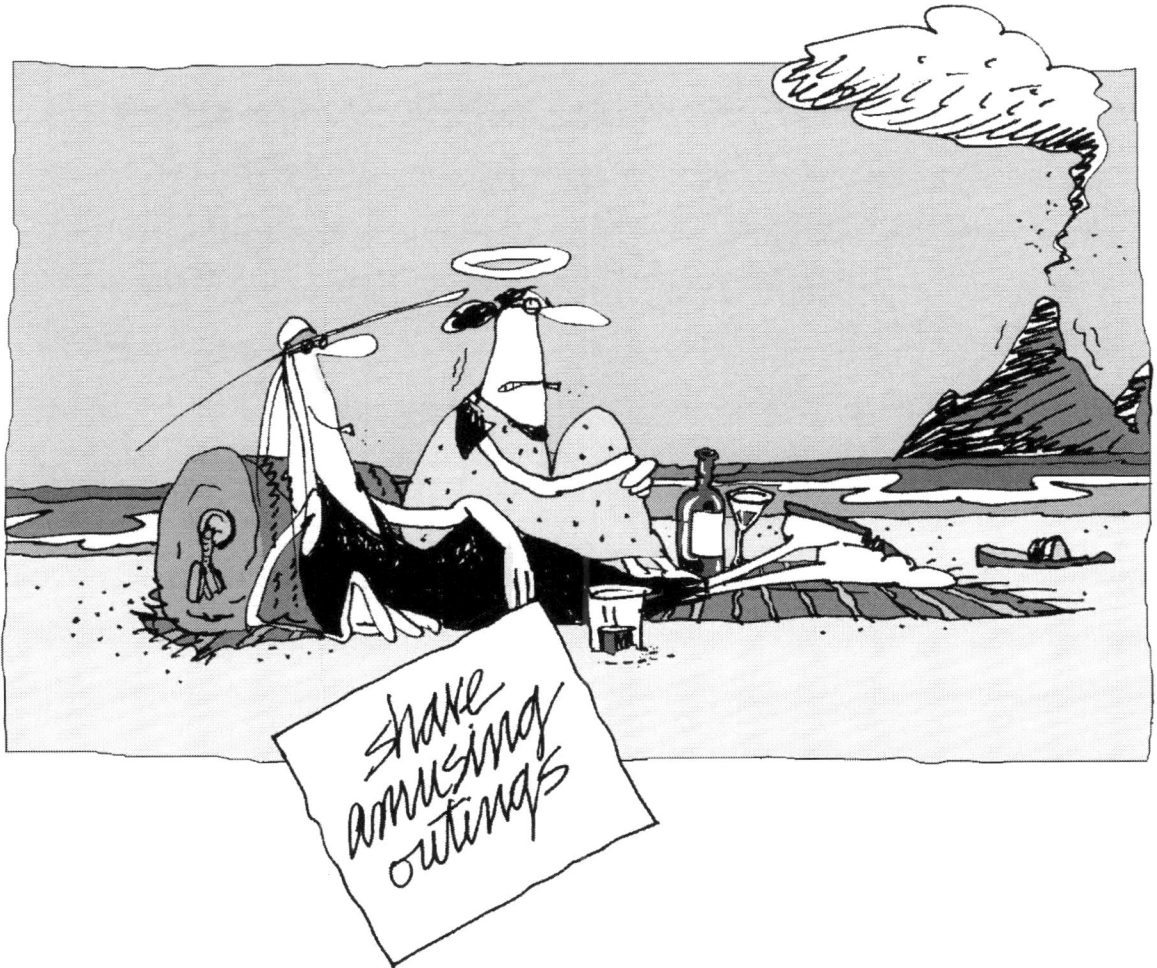

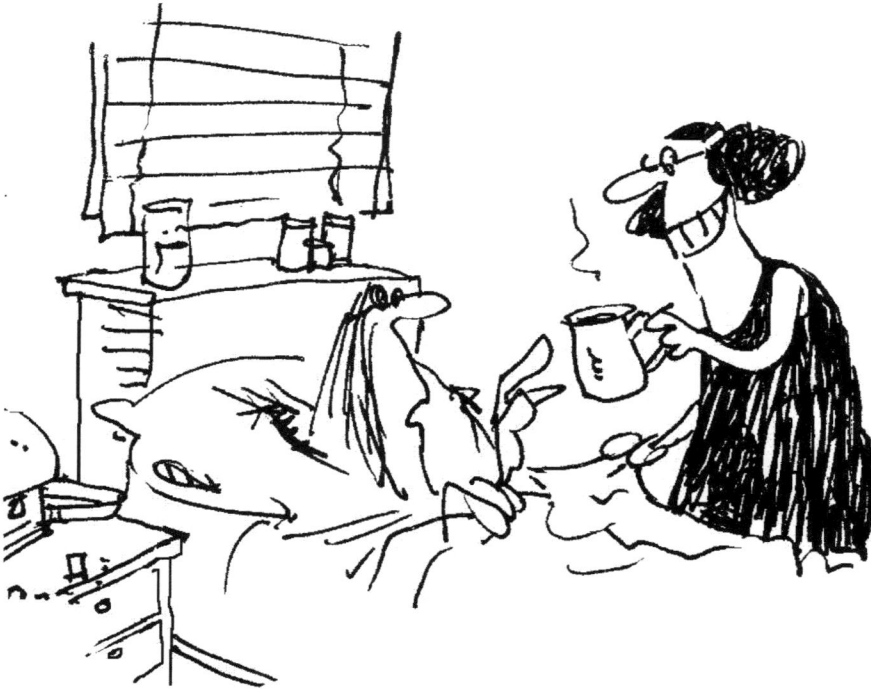

Great Travel Saints are born not made

Traveling alone is possible, but it's way easier (and far more fun) with someone else. What you want is a god, goddess or saint. Someone who'll put up with your occasional whining, bring you food when you're too ill to go out, find your meds when you can't remember your name . . . and who still enjoys sharing a room with you if necessary.

Maybe you have a person in your life that loves you and loves to travel with you, in which case you're lucky and can ignore the rest of this chapter.

Some might think that an energetic companion would be a good idea as high energy people are much valued in our society. But in the search for a Travel Saint, high energy is best avoided. What you want is a laid-back companion. One who doesn't mind sitting in a café for an hour watching the passing scene, one who prefers reading to hiking, one who has no interest in long-distance walking and is never averse to a little rest.

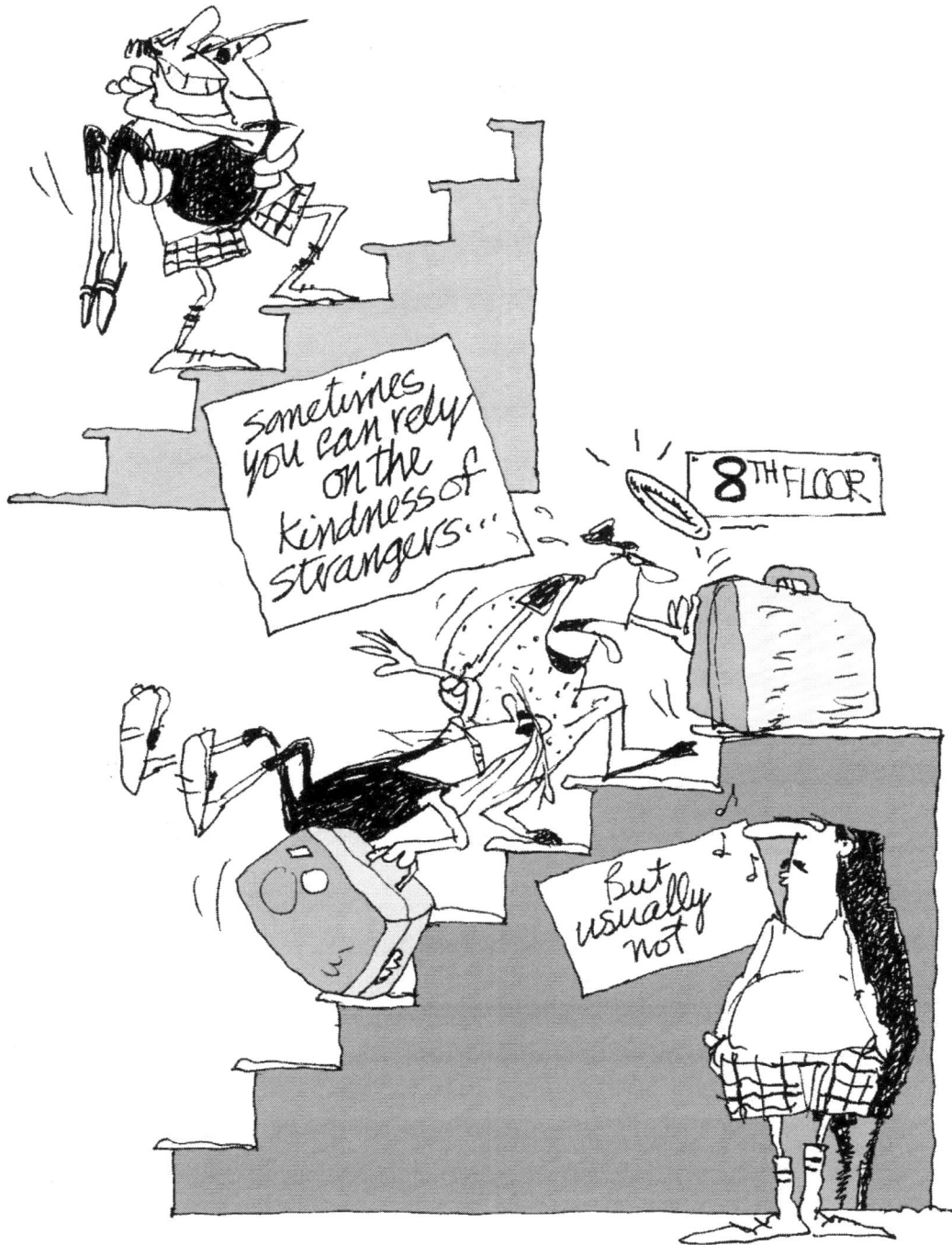

If you're in the enviable position of being able to choose your travel companion from several equally wonderful people, certain traits make one person a more suitable Travel Saint than another.

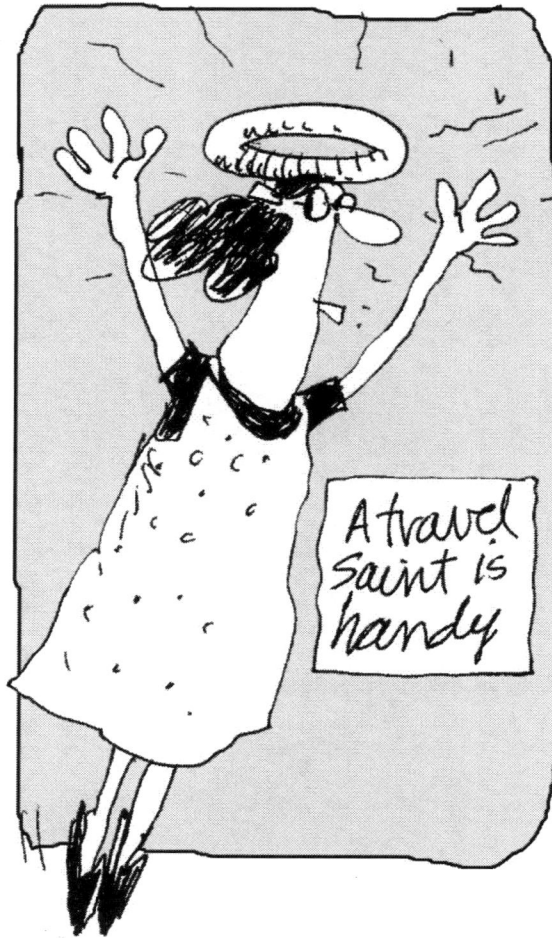

The main requirement, obviously, is empathy. But all of your candidates may have that.

Another factor is adaptability — those of us with chronic pain are not always reliable when it comes to plans. If the pain is too great, we might have to pass on something we really wanted to do (and planned to do with our friend). And that sometimes leaves the travel companion at loose ends. Traveling with someone who is too rigid to adapt well to last-minute change can be problematic.

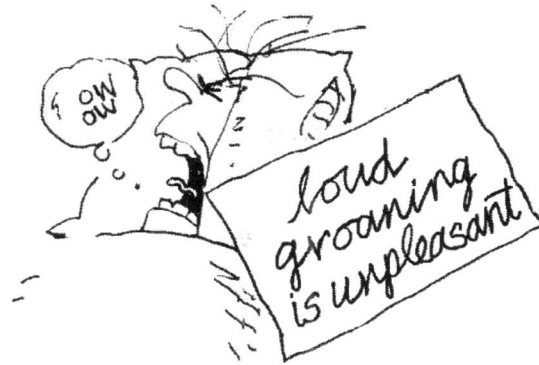

The reason for choosing the more lethargic partner should be pretty clear to anyone living with chronic pain. You're probably not a ball of fire 100% of the time. Why wear yourself to a string trying to keep up with your travel partner or constantly feel as if you're holding him or her back?

Unless, of course, this terribly energetic pal is completely in tune with your slower pace, has no problem at all striking out on his or her own, and you love them to pieces. In which case, lucky you—travel together by all means!

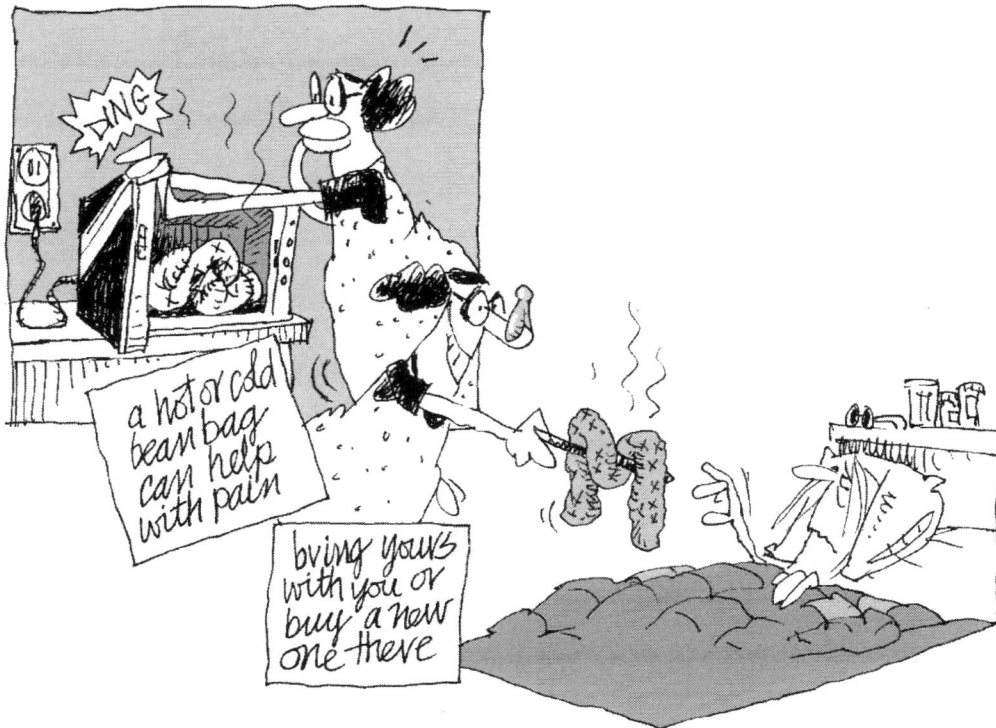

No matter which Travel Saint accompanies you into the Great Unknown, you'll need a little help at times. Ask for it. Your pal is probably not a mind reader, already understands you'll be in serious pain sometimes and is absolutely willing to do whatever is necessary to help you.

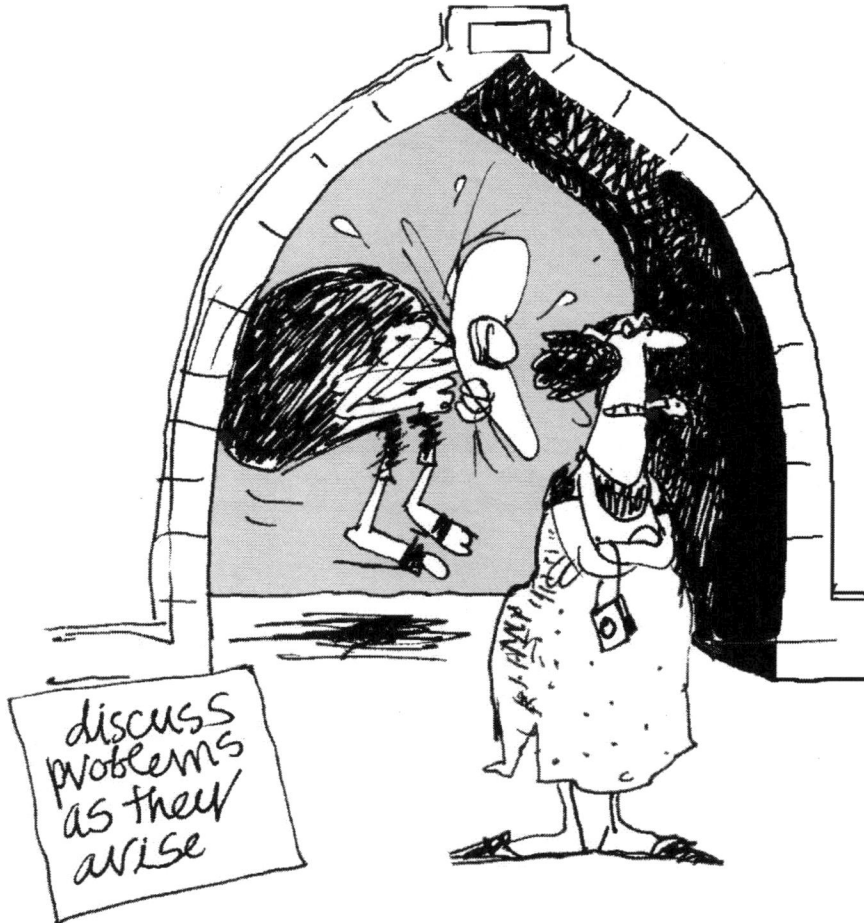

Although you won't whine on endlessly, and will do your best to keep to whatever schedule you've made together, it's still much better to let your friend know it's time for you to rest than to keep on keeping on when you really shouldn't. You'll end up in some kind of crisis, and the Travel Saint will have to earn his or her halo by picking up the pieces. Better to speak up earlier and avoid a lot of pain for both of you.

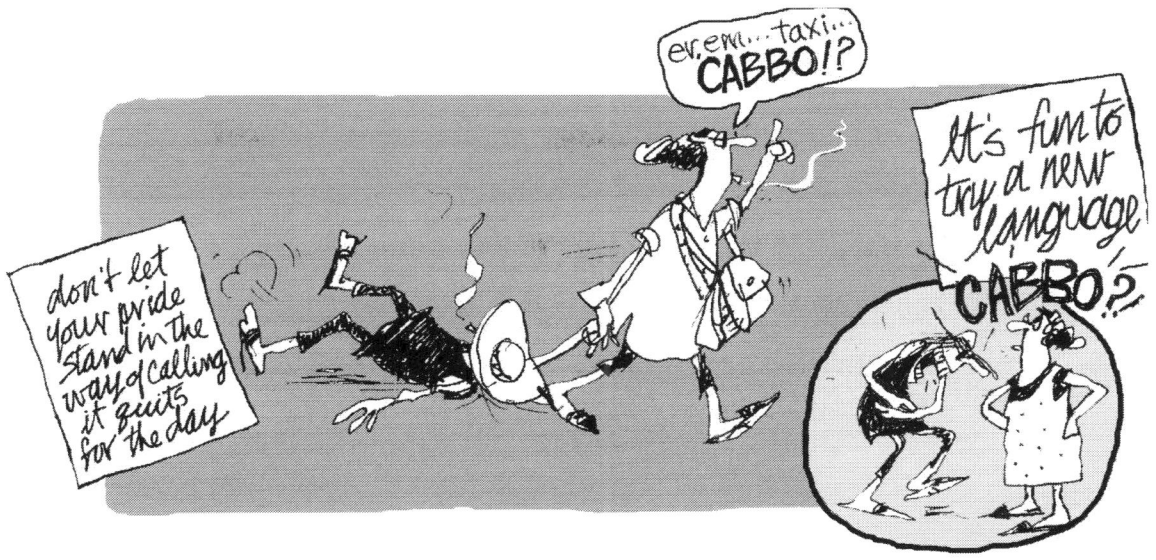

It's difficult to allow yourself the luxury of showing pain, especially if you've lived most of your life attempting to keep it to yourself. But this whole business of traveling with someone who knows about your condition is one of trust: you trust them enough to expose your vulnerability, and they trust you enough to know you won't take advantage of their sympathy. It's a delicate balance and a rare, wonderfully mutual relationship — but so is great friendship.

You're very lucky to have each other.

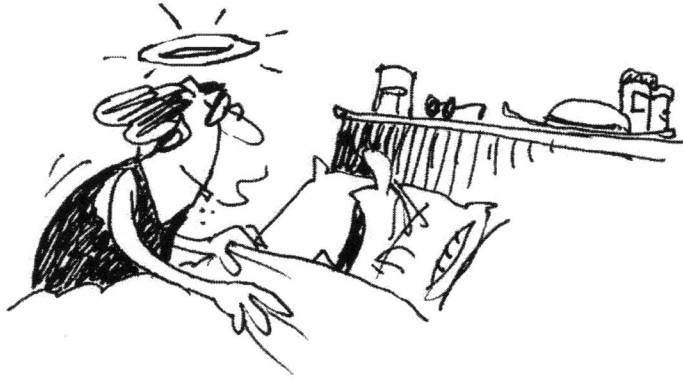

Chapter 3
WHAT TO TAKE

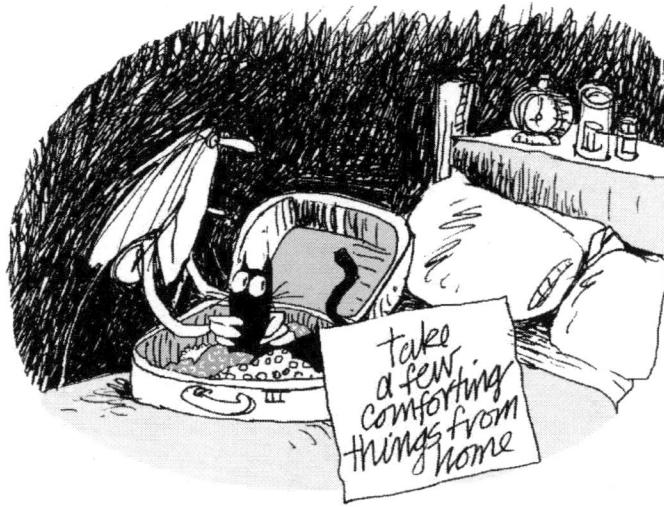

For the traveler with chronic pain, less is not always more

Maybe you've listened to all that travel advice about only taking one small bag. Don't despair! That travel advice is not for the chronically afflicted. I don't know about you, but except for weekend getaways, I've never been able to manage with only one small bag. The traveling meds alone practically take up a whole suitcase.

In my experience, it's much better to bring all the things you'll need:

Passport and visa (if a visa is required).

If you need a special pillow, bring it.

If you need ice packs, bring them.

If you need particular loungewear simply because it provides comfort, pack it.

You get the idea.

Medication

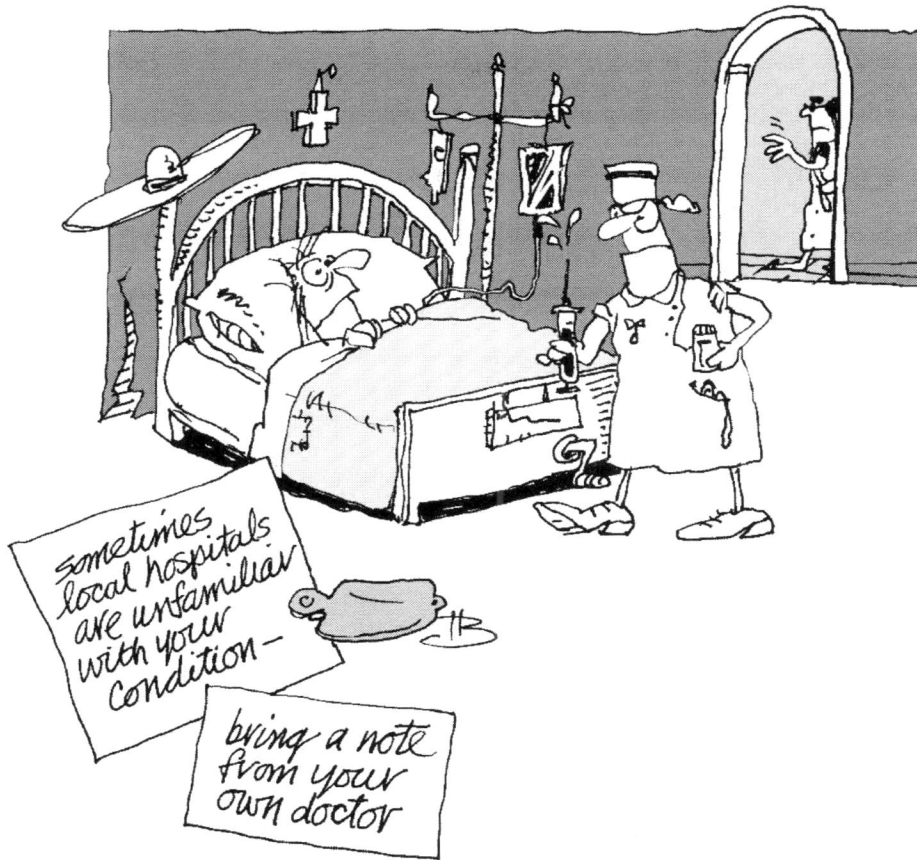

sometimes local hospitals are unfamiliar with your condition—

bring a note from your own doctor

Make an appointment with your doctor a few weeks before you go to discuss your travel plans:

Length of time you'll be away

Destination

Projected pain levels

Vaccinations or shots you'll need before leaving.

If you're going away for long enough, you should fill an extra prescription or two. Getting replacement drugs in another country almost always means seeing a doctor, and sometimes, language problems aside, it's difficult convincing a doctor who has never seen you before that you actually do suffer from chronic pain — it isn't as obvious as some other disabilities. With so many drug addicts masquerading as people in chronic pain, you can't blame doctors for being wary.

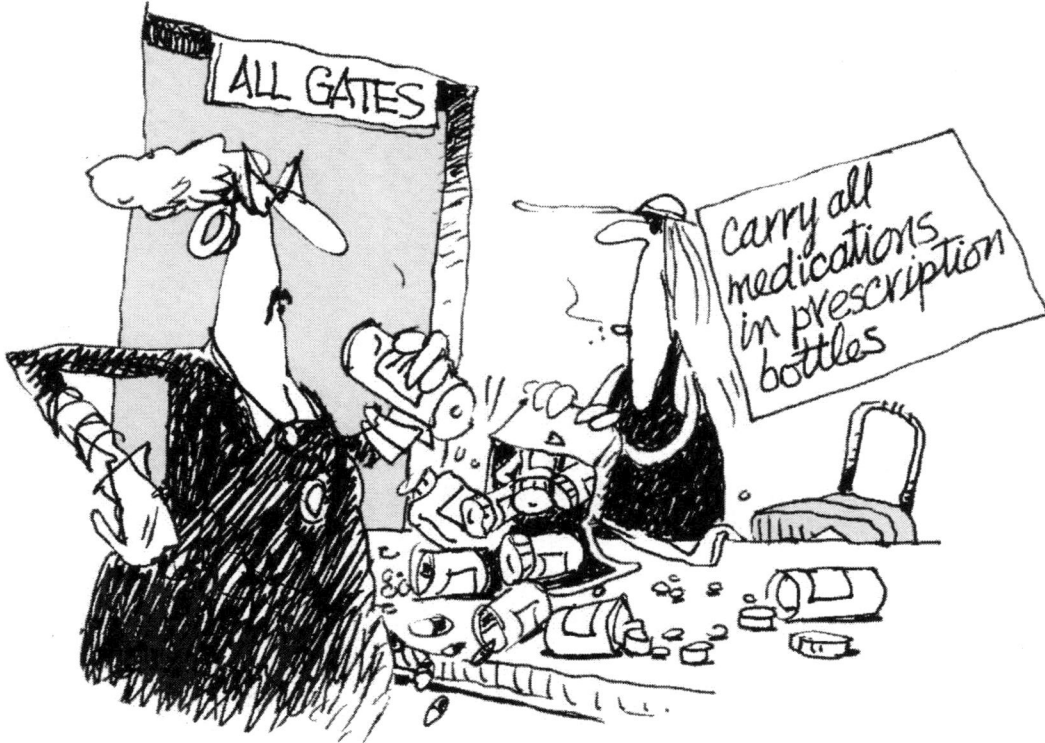

If you're worried about carrying a lot of narcotics through customs, have your doctor write a short note on his or her prescription pad, outlining your condition and listing your medications. You probably won't need it, but it's reassuring to have just in case.

Never pack your meds in checked baggage. Always carry them on the plane with you. Luggage gets lost and you definitely don't want to be far, far from home without your prescriptions.

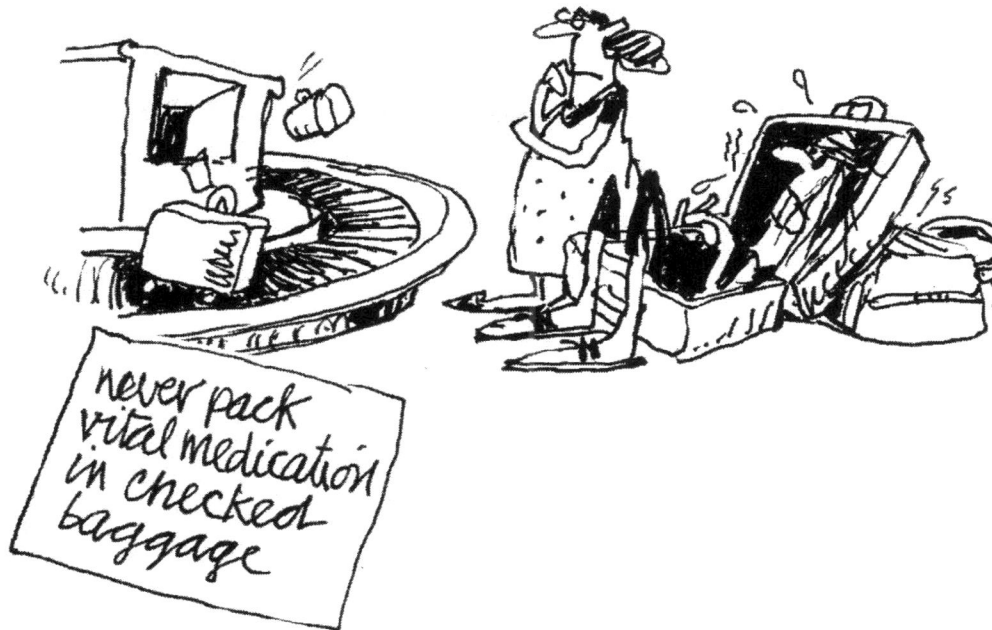

never pack vital medication in checked baggage

You could also leave a prescription at your pharmacy or with a friend so that if your meds are lost or stolen, they could express deliver them to you if you're in one place long enough.

A lot of medications take up a lot of room and because of all your special requirements, it's almost impossible to travel with only a carry-on bag. Bring what you need.

Cash

It's no longer necessary to carry large amounts of cash or traveler's checks. You can access your accounts almost everywhere at ATMs or banks or just use a credit card most of the time. Do get a small amount of money in the currency of the country you're going to for airport spending and transport to your hotel.

Bags

Most travel advisors say pack light and take very little with you. It's great advice because you don't have to hoist and haul your endless baggage everywhere you go, but for people who have chronic pain, life is a little different. You have particular needs, and if you don't bring certain items with you, you'll either have more discomfort than you already experience or you'll spend valuable—and stressful—time hunting them down in a foreign land where, for instance, they might never have heard of a microwaveable beanbag.

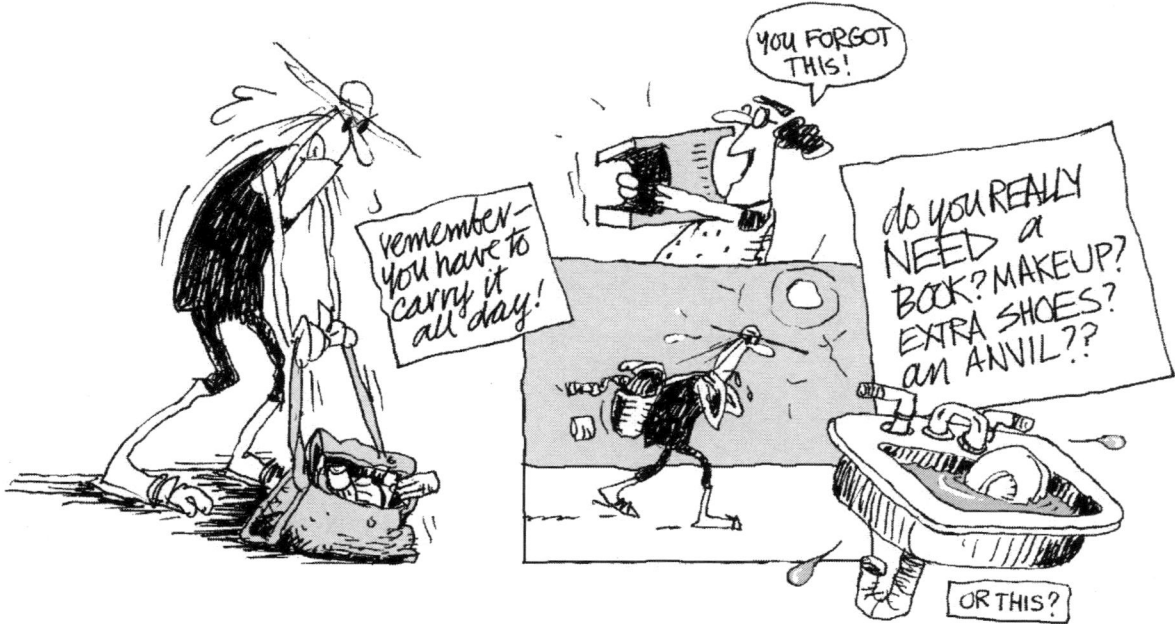

Use wheeled suitcases, preferably hard-shell ones with four wheels. They're easier to push and they can act as a seat or even a table in an emergency or long line. And if you're only going to one destination, moving two suitcases around won't be that hard.

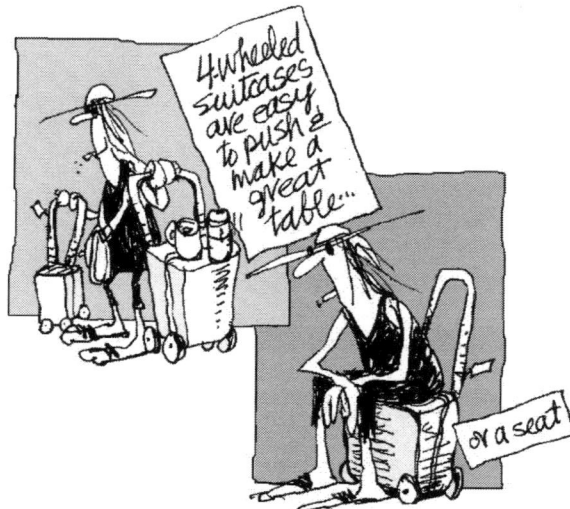

Do try to keep to one checked bag and one carry-on (and a purse or man-bag). Anything else is way too difficult to deal with in transit.

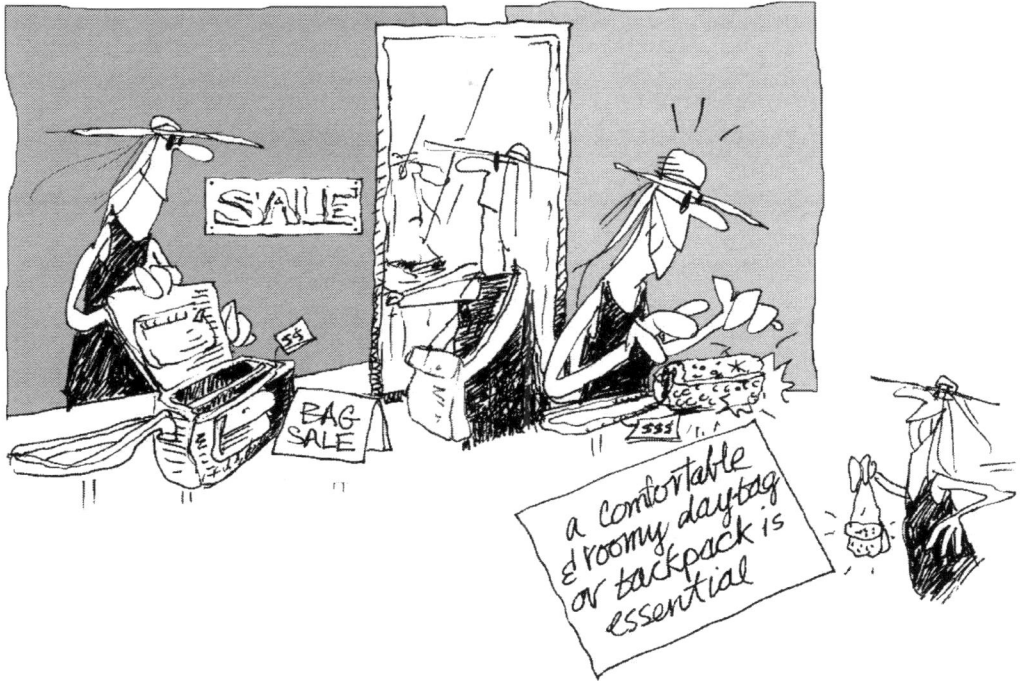

a comfortable & roomy daybag or backpack is essential

Clothes

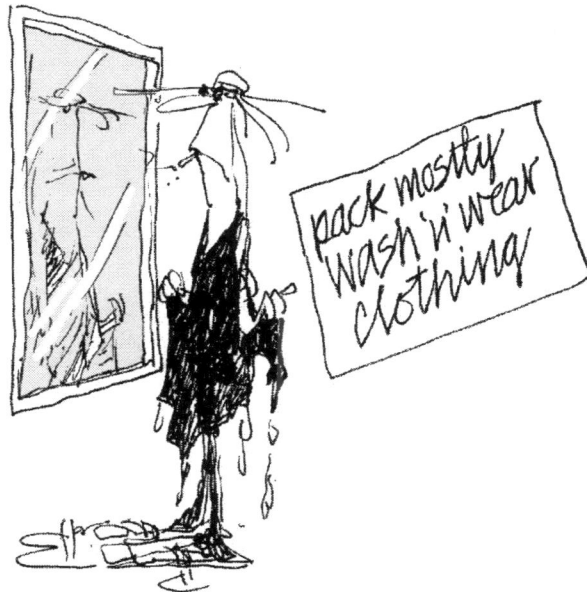

pack mostly wash 'n' wear clothing

Almost certainly you'll only want about half the clothes you think you'll need. Be ruthless with clothing, shoes and accessories. Make more room for your pain meds.

If absolutely necessary, you can always buy another bag while you're away to bring things home, but I would advise leaving a little room in your suitcase for purchases. An extra bag is a headache...and you're already in enough pain.

Tablets and Smart Phones

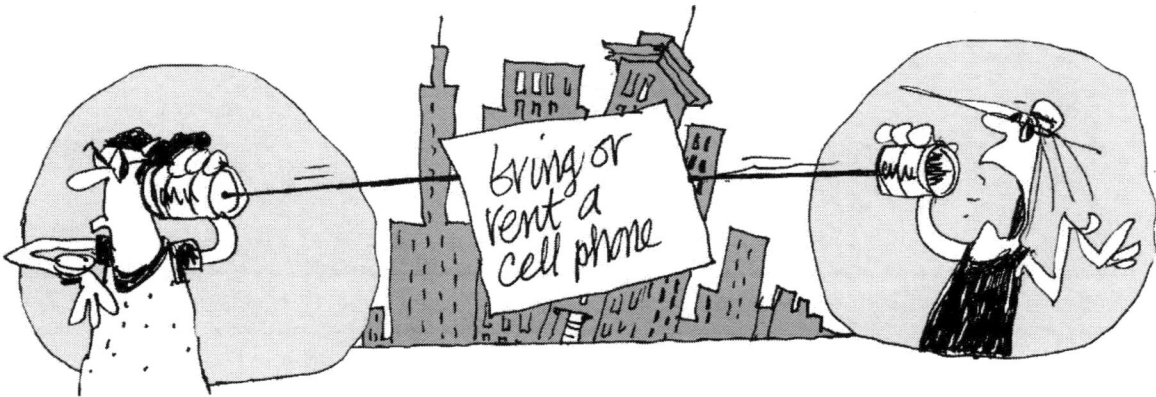

Tablets and smart phones with Internet access are wonderful travel tools. They can store as many books as you'll want to read, plus music, videos, movies and even maps. One of these devices will take the place of all the guides, books and maps you used to need. You can download any number of apps to help you understand the places you're visiting, and even aid with language and interpreting basic things like menus and signs. E-mail lets you keep in touch with everyone back home, and if you're traveling with a friend, you can find each other easily by phone or text if you're accidentally separated.

Do look into a foreign-travel plan with your phone provider before you go, or if you have an unlocked device, use a local SIM card (usually less than $10.00) — much cheaper than paying exorbitant long-distance charges on every call.

Things I Like to Take

Each of us has his or her own needs, but I've found the following things very useful:

Refillable water bottle

Light-weight shawl

Folding cane if you need one

And a few other specially made travel items if you think you'll need them, e.g., amazing travel stores even have fabulous, crush-proof straw hats.

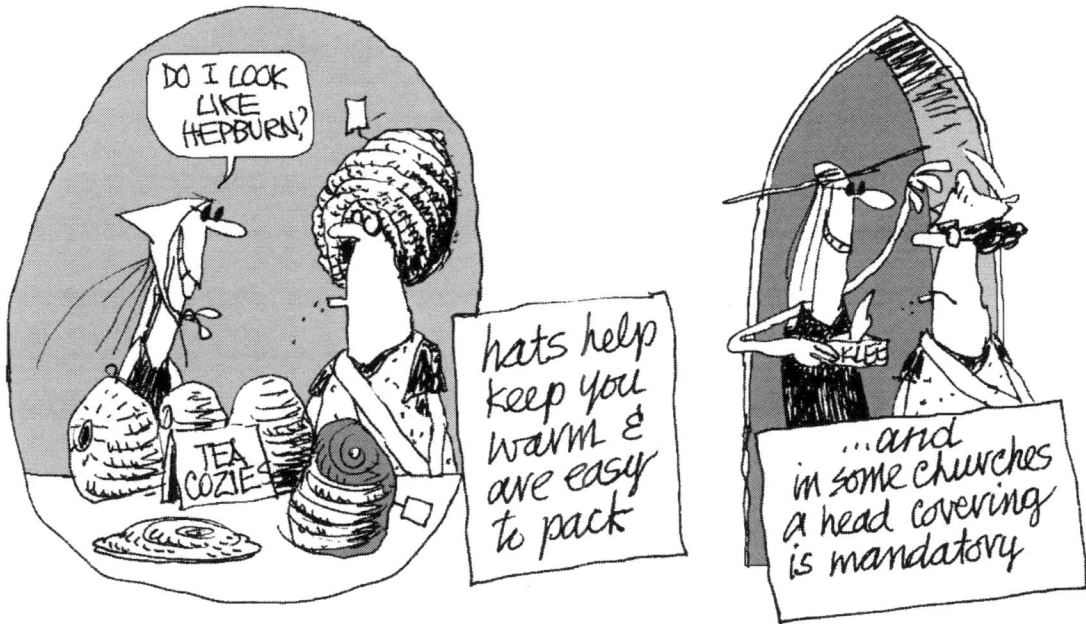

Buy and take what you need and what you can afford. But don't get ridiculous—less is more in the travel-gadget department.

The Three Rules in Travel

Comfort, comfort, comfort—your comfort is the most important thing to keep in mind when packing. Living anywhere other than your home will mean a certain amount of strangeness. Having your comforts met as much as possible will ensure a much happier trip.

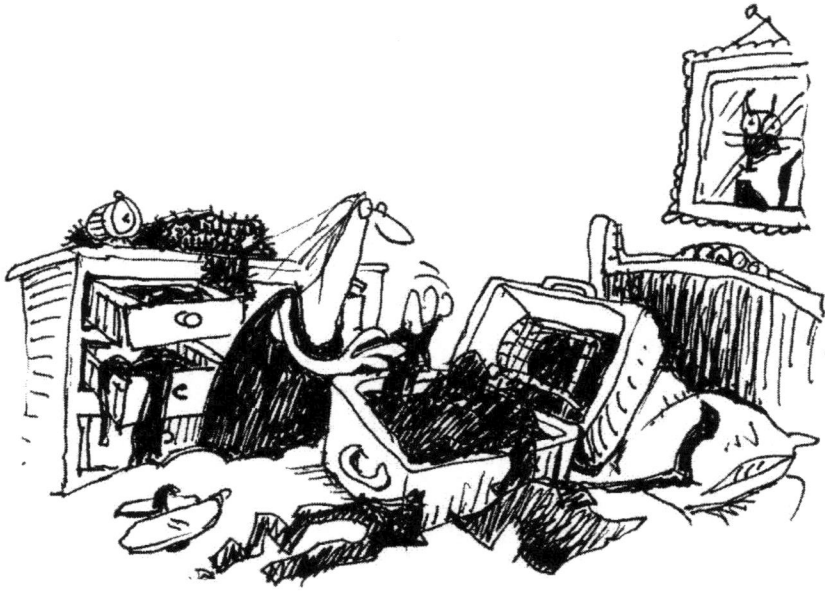

Chapter 4
GETTING THERE

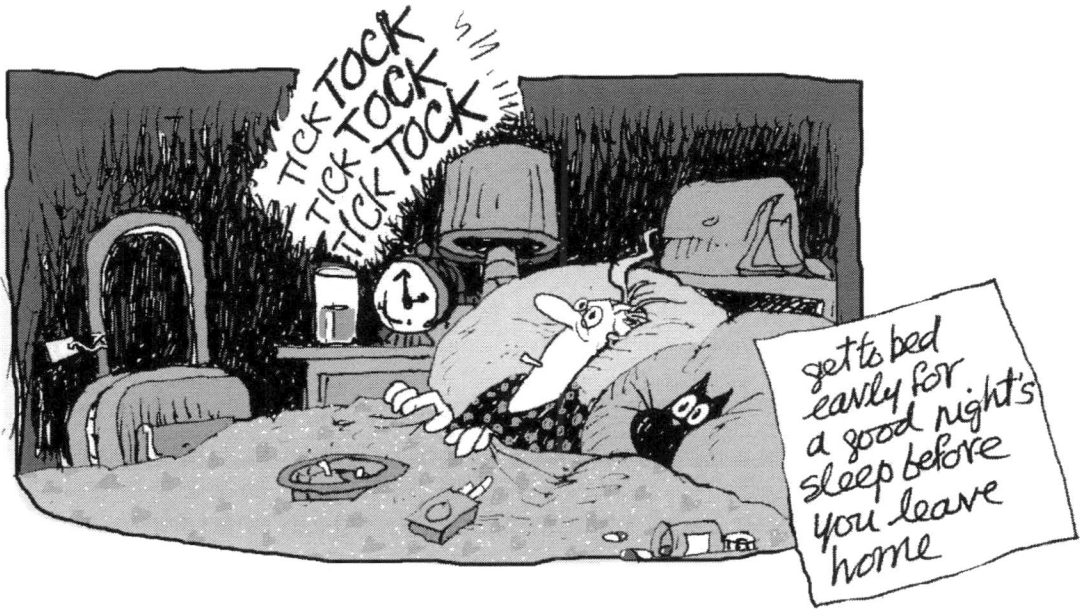

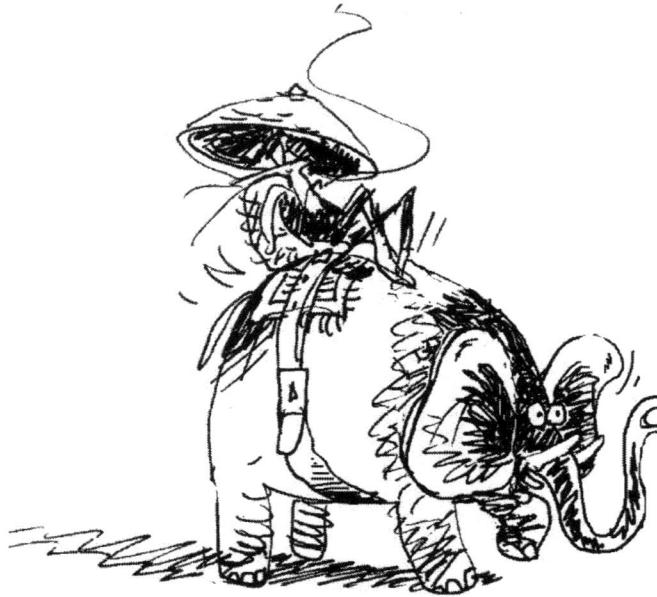

If getting there is difficult, overmedicating will make it more so

In my experience, unless you're on a cruise, getting there is NOT half the fun. In fact, it's almost none of the fun. And even with a cruise, you still have to get to wherever the cruise leaves from. Of course getting there in an RV or similarly equipped van is perfect — you leave from home and travel with a bed and kitchen. Unfortunately, you can't RV everywhere (even if you're lucky enough to have one). Airplanes, large ships, houseboats and sleeper trains are all reasonably comfortable. Backpacking, camping tours, buses, camels and whatnot, not so much.

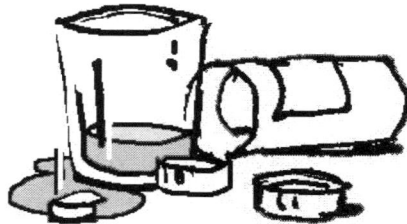

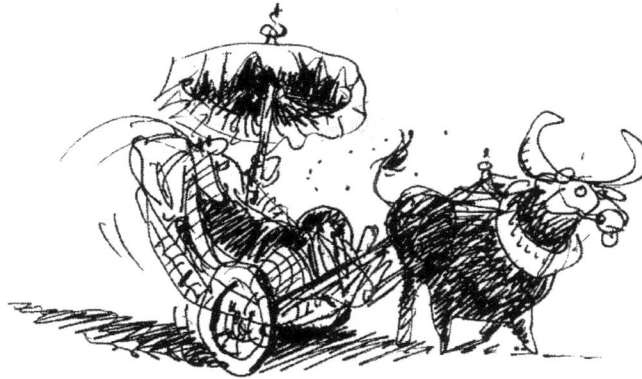

Sometimes even 'comfortable' modes of transit are trying for those of us with chronic pain. The final destination IS worth it, but the more prepared you are, the less difficult — and painful — it will be.

Be discerning and, above all, be honest with yourself when planning your trip. What might be exciting and fun for normal people could be excruciating for you.

Let's say you decide to travel by wagon train. Best case, you'll be in constant pain. Worst case, you'll drop out and find the nearest airport. Either way, it's probably a waste of money, a waste of effort and absolutely not fun.

Before you book any kind of offbeat travel, imagine yourself actually taking the trip:

Will it be terribly uncomfortable given your pain?

Will there be far too much walking involved?

Will sleeping be difficult or uncomfortable?

Will temperature extremes affect your pain?

Will you be able to keep up with others?

Once you've honestly pictured yourself taking the trip, if you think you can do it, by all means do. But if you're fairly sure your condition will make the trip far too painful, rethink your travel plans. People who suffer from chronic pain can't do absolutely everything — but travel options abound. There will almost always be another way of getting to where you want to go.

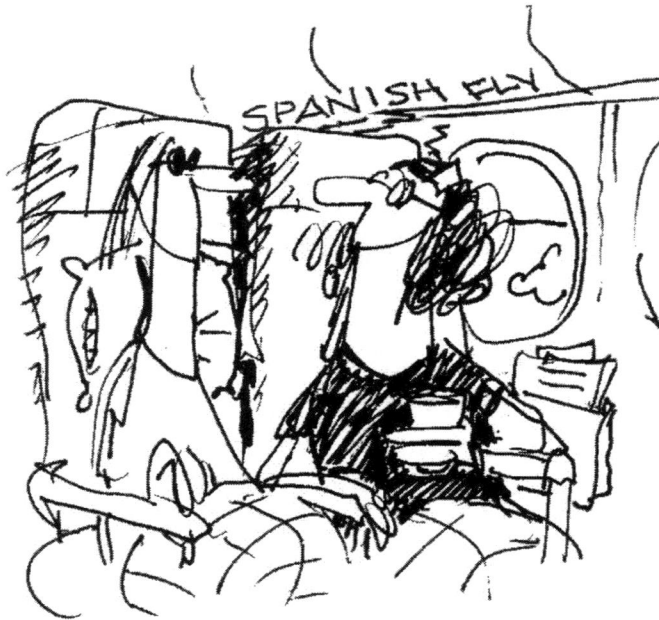

For the purposes of this guide, I'm assuming you have enough money to travel nicely but not enough to travel first class everywhere you go.

If you're in the backpack/hostel group (even though cursed with chronic pain), if you're young and adventurous, and if you have an understanding, patient traveling companion, why not give it a try? But be advised, it will be very difficult sometimes. You might want to bring enough money for a night in a hotel now and then just to recover.

For the rest of us who aren't packing our lives on our back, we can do things that will help enormously with the discomfort of travel.

Arranging the Trip

If your computer skills aren't up to booking online, travel agents are still a good alternative to the do-it-yourself holiday. Explain your specific needs to the agent and leave the intricacies of travel planning up to them. They're usually able to get good deals and often have personal knowledge of your destination.

If your destination is far from home and your journey isn't direct but involves changing conveyances, consider stopping over en route. For anyone with chronic pain, it's often well worth adding a day or two to the journey, to rest and recuperate before continuing to your final destination.

Before you even leave home, book a hotel at your journey's end. If you're in a lot of pain on arrival, the first thing you'll want to do is get to a comfortable bed, take some pain meds, and rest or sleep for a while (sometimes a long while) till you have more or less adjusted to any time changes and are ready to hit the town.

If you can, try to pick an arrival time to coincide with the check-in time at your hotel (usually mid-afternoon). You don't want to spend dazed hours hauling your suitcases around a foreign locale till your room is ready. However, most hotels will store your bags for you and you can sit in the lobby or find a nearby restaurant.

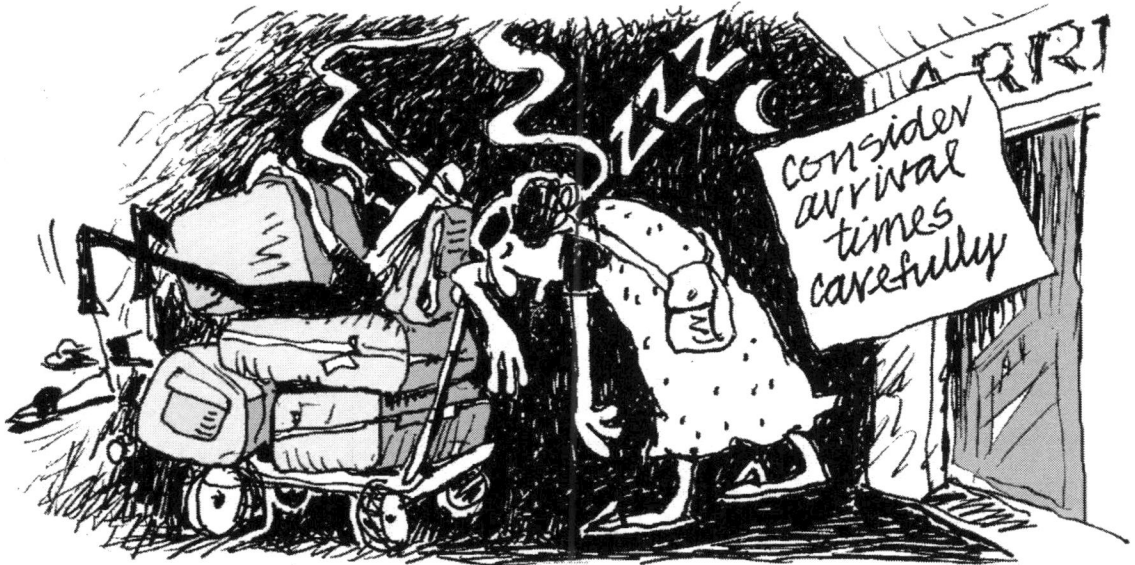

Waiting

To get to your dream destination, you'll probably need to travel according to the schedule of your transportation provider, and you'll have to walk and wait, and walk and wait . . . just to get to the boarding gate. Once at the gate, you'll have to wait and wait, and line-up and wait...

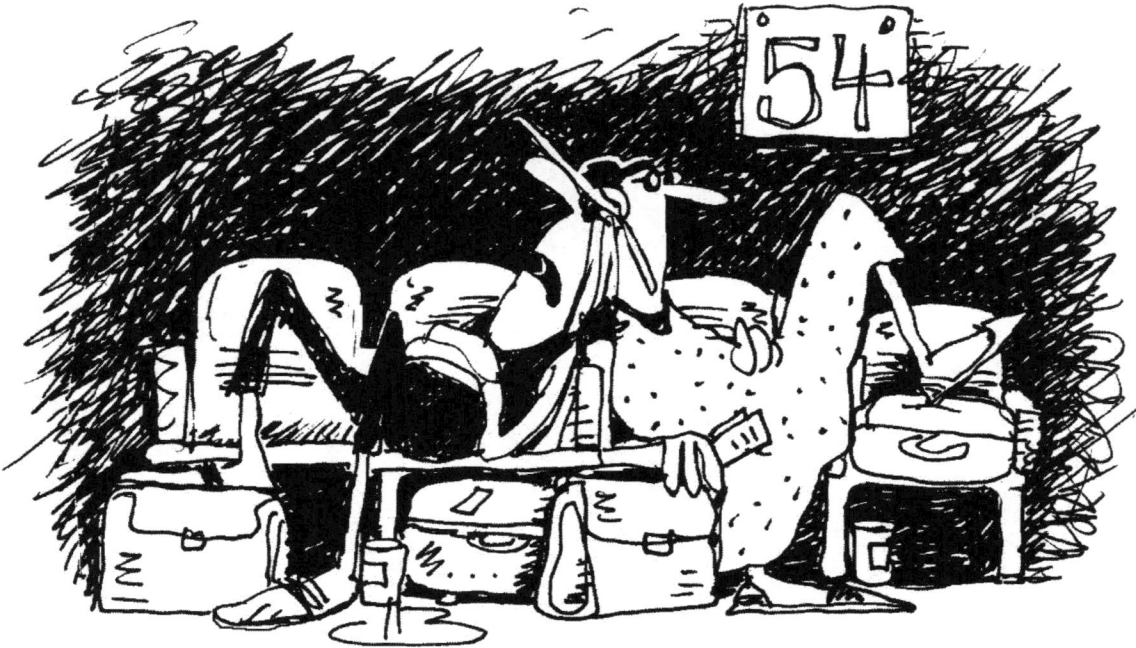

In fact, one of the most potentially pain-inducing parts of travel — and certainly the most boring — is waiting. It seems everywhere you go, no matter what mode of transport you use, some amount of waiting is involved. This usually means sitting on a hard plastic chair for hours but often also means standing in line for far too long. If your traveling companion doesn't mind too much, let her wait in line for both of you. You can fetch coffee.

Some of the tips in the section (below) on air travel will apply to other forms of transportation as well.

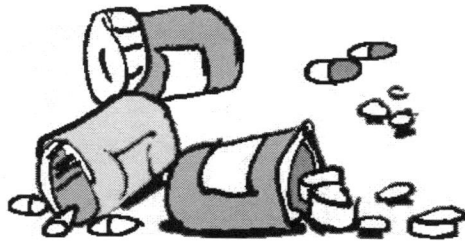

Air Travel

Many airlines will let you book a wheelchair or space on an in-terminal golf cart. Just be sure to book ahead (at both ends) since this kind of transportation is often at a premium. If you have trouble standing in line, use the pre-boarding option to get on the plane a little before the rest of the passengers.

Be careful what you eat or drink before boarding a plane. The healthier the choices you make in the airport lounge, the less discomfort you'll experience on board. Drink water or juice, eat salads or light meals. Heavy food sits like a stone in your innards when you're inactive.

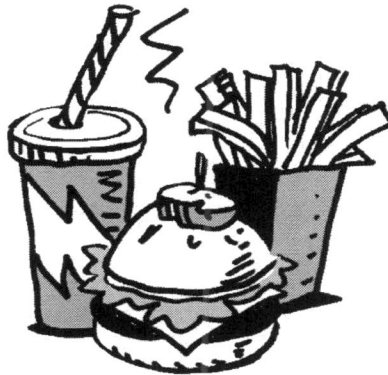

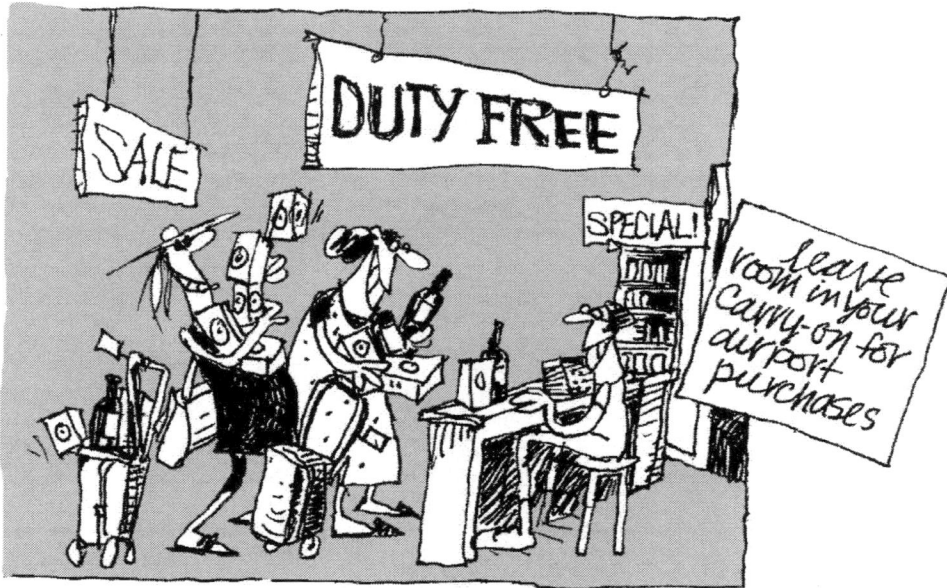

Take some healthy snacks: nuts, trail mix, whatever you enjoy. And if you're traveling by plane, on many flights these days you must bring your own meals or suffer the consequences of in-flight choices (although full meals are usually available on overnight flights). Just remember that almost all airline rules prohibit carrying liquids on board. Buying what you need AFTER you've gone through security is the safest plan.

And don't get carried away with the in-flight wines and liquors. Not only will they dehydrate you, but mixing pain meds with alcohol can have serious consequences. Besides, you don't want your Travel Saint to have to carry you off the plane.

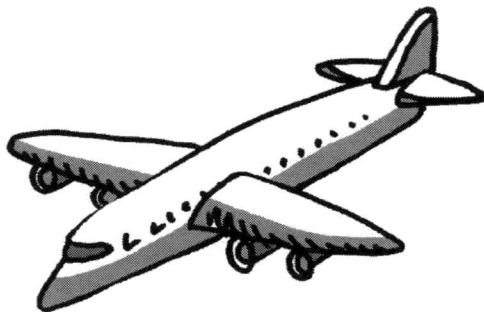

OWww!

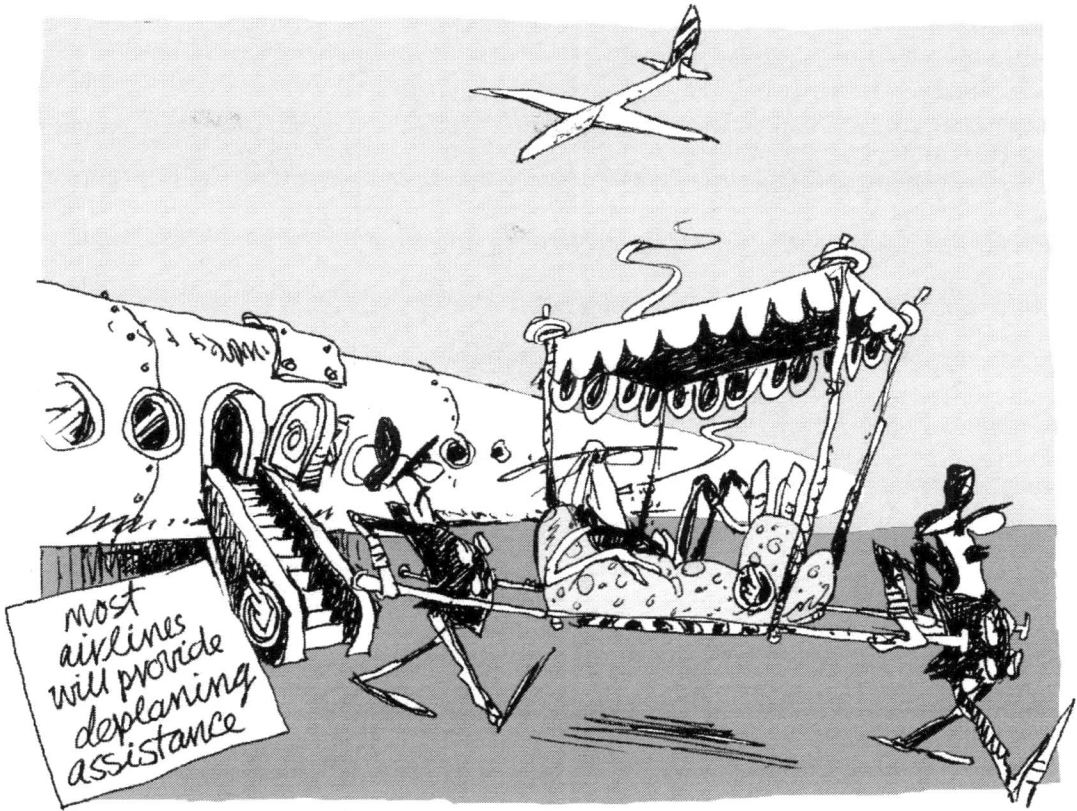

most airlines will provide deplaning assistance

If your pain has peaked, wait till others have deplaned before leaving

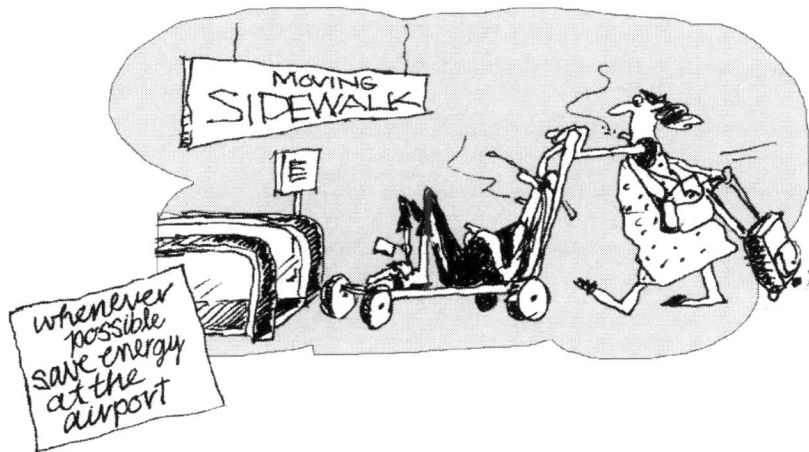

MOVING SIDEWALK

E

whenever possible save energy at the airport

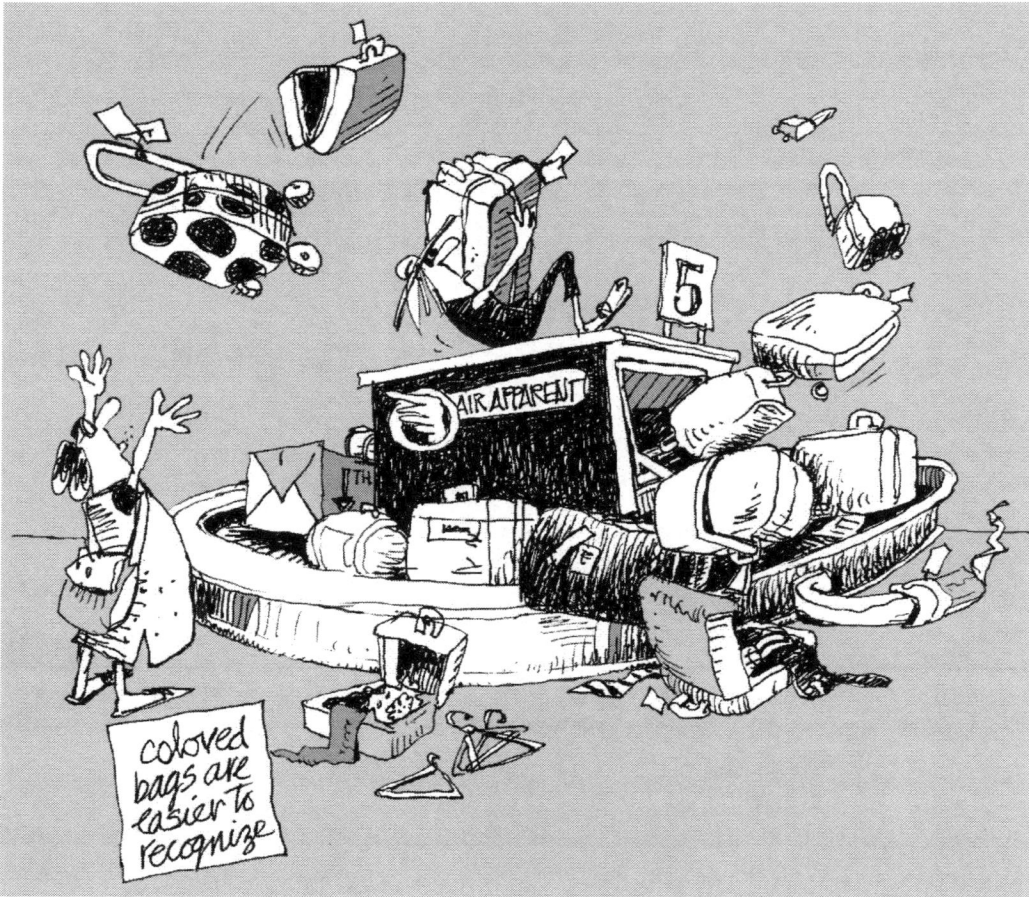

As mentioned elsewhere in this guide, THE most important things to carry while traveling are your medications. Put all of them, in their original prescription bottles (to make it easier at security), in your carry-on bag just in case your checked suitcases get lost for a while.

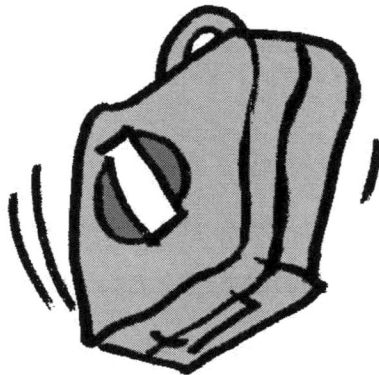

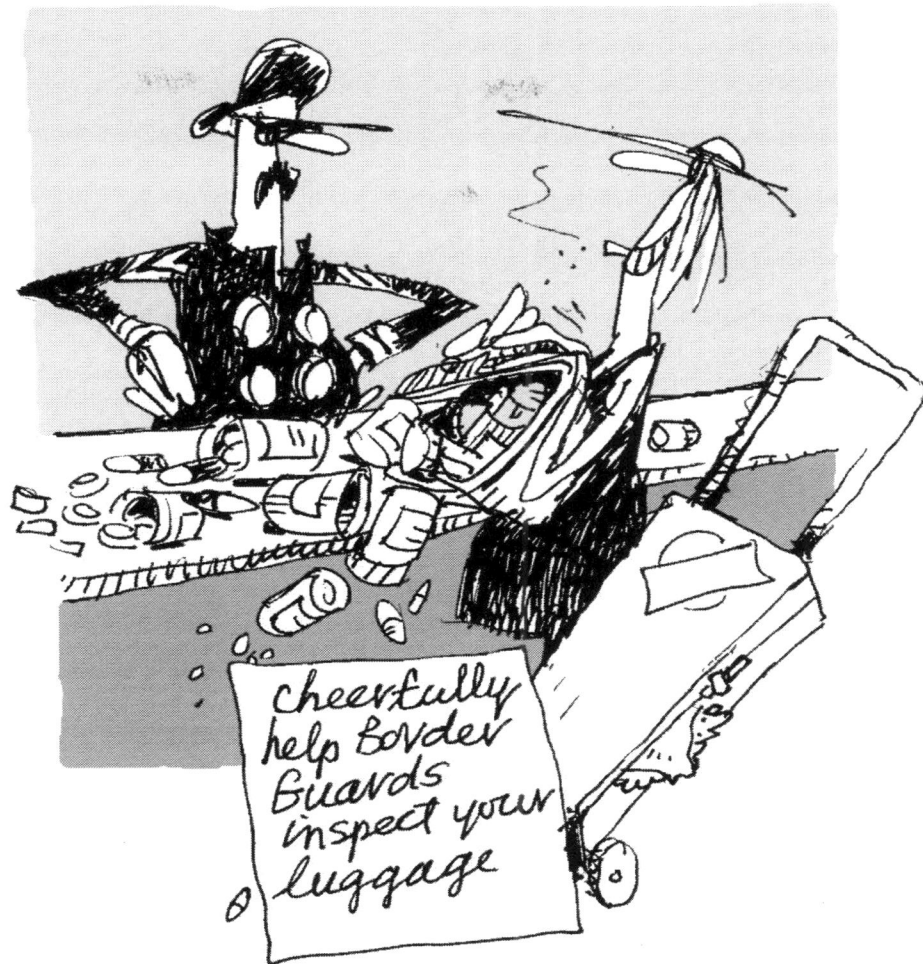

cheerfully help Border Guards inspect your luggage

Remember to keep track of the pills you're taking. With time changes and the weird, twilight feeling of being out-of-time on long trips, it's easy to forget you've already taken pain medication or sleeping pills and take a second dose too soon. Keep track in a small notebook or consult your Travel Saint, who likely remembers more than you do at this point.

A pillow is a must for your neck, the small of your back or anywhere else you need support. Blow-up pillows fit in your carry-on, but I prefer the preformed ones. They're firm, covered in soft fabric and major bonus, you don't have to blow them up! However, they are bulky. If you can't jam it into your bag, wander through the terminal with a pillow hanging from your neck—you absolutely won't be alone.

A thin shawl or lightweight sweater is a great comfort when napping or sleeping in transit. They provide warmth yet still pack into a small space, and are much more comforting than the tiny blanket provided by airlines. Both the shawl and the sweater will serve you in good stead at your destination if you need extra warmth at night.

For those bothered by light or sound, eye masks and earplugs are mandatory. A pair of folding slippers is very useful when spending a long time sitting down in a pressurized environment. Take your shoes off, don your slip-ons, let your feet swell if they must, and pad around in comfort. Your feet will thank you.

And do remember to get up and walk around periodically during a long flight—it helps your circulation when you've been sitting in one position for too long. Some might also find compression socks a boon to circulation.

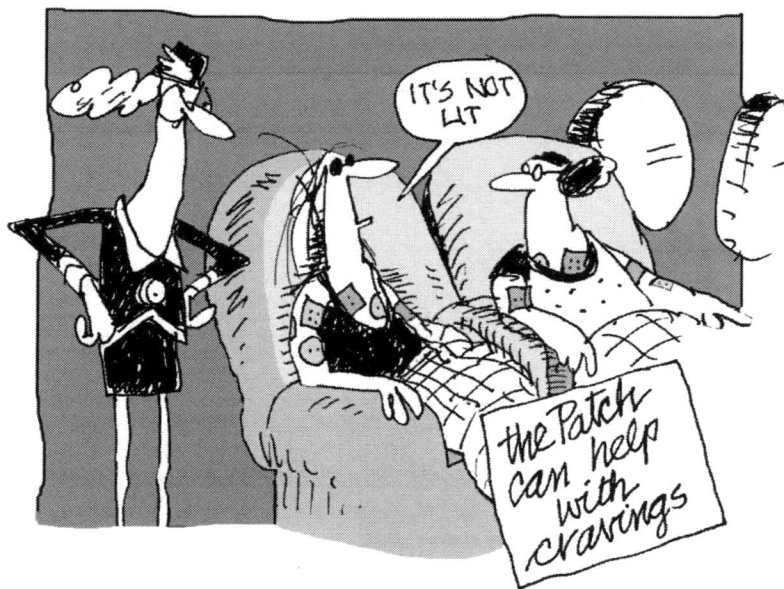

For die-hard smokers: nicotine patches, gum, or the fabulous electronic cigarettes (a.k.a. e-cigarettes) can allay cravings

A small thermos or collapsible bottle full of water is a handy travel item. Often your thirst precedes the drinks trolley. It's much 'greener' than buying bottles of water, and worth the space it takes up, as you'll use it everywhere while touring. (A shoulder strap for the thermos is a good investment.)

However you get there, be prepared to combat some of the discomfort. Travel with your basic needs in your personal bag, sleep as much as possible, if possible, and arrive tired, but reasonably well. Get a cab to your hotel, sleep till you feel human again, and let the fun begin.

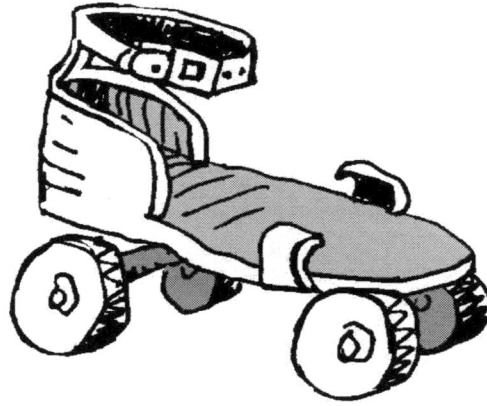

Chapter 5
WHERE TO STAY

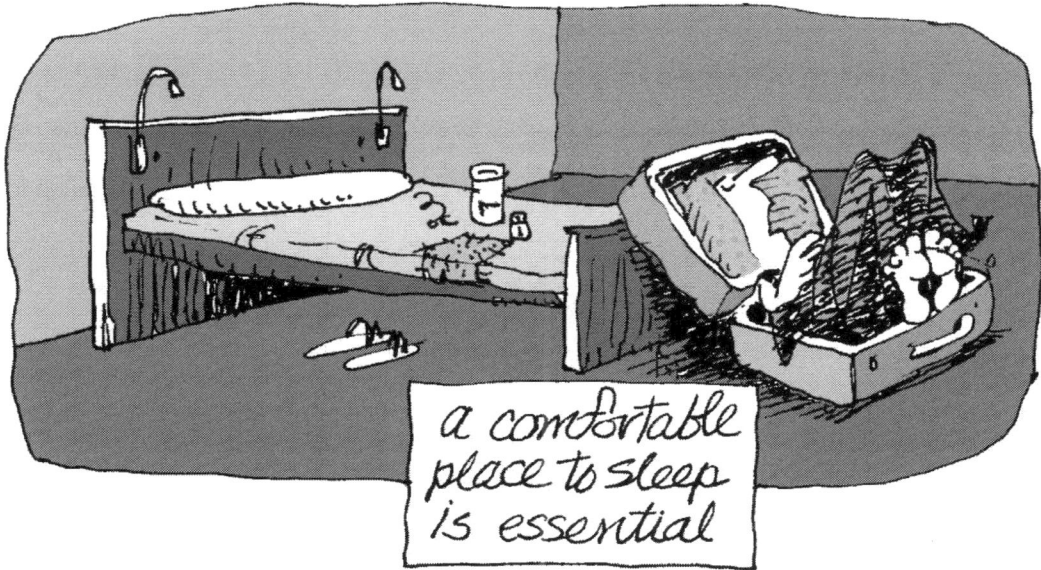

a comfortable place to sleep is essential

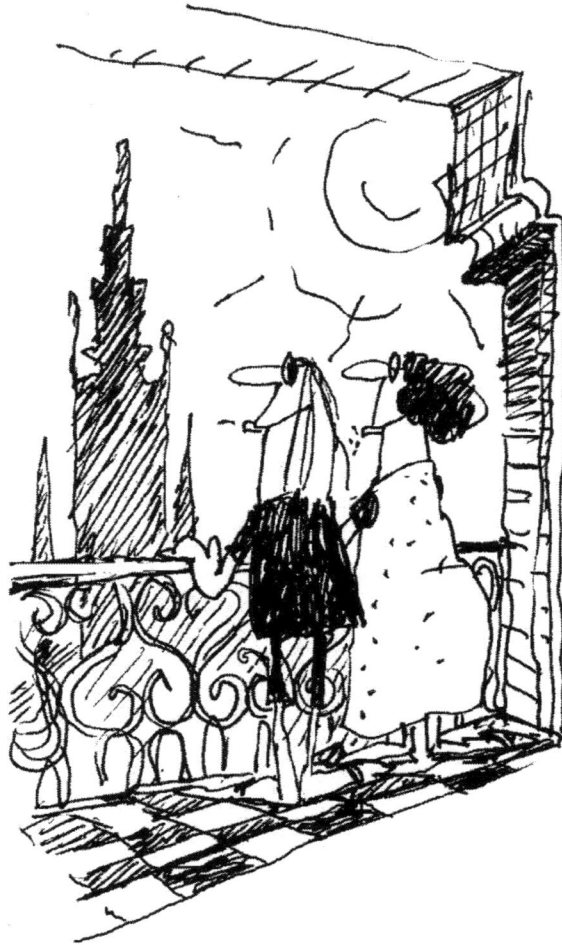

Before booking, make sure lodgings will meet all your requirements

If your budget is unlimited, skip this chapter—hell, skip the book, and hire a travel nurse! But if your funds are somewhat more modest, read on.

The right choice of accommodation can't be overemphasized; it can make or break a holiday. Anyone who suffers from chronic pain needs a clean, airy, comfortable place to stay. And a good bed.

But these are not the only considerations.

My Faves

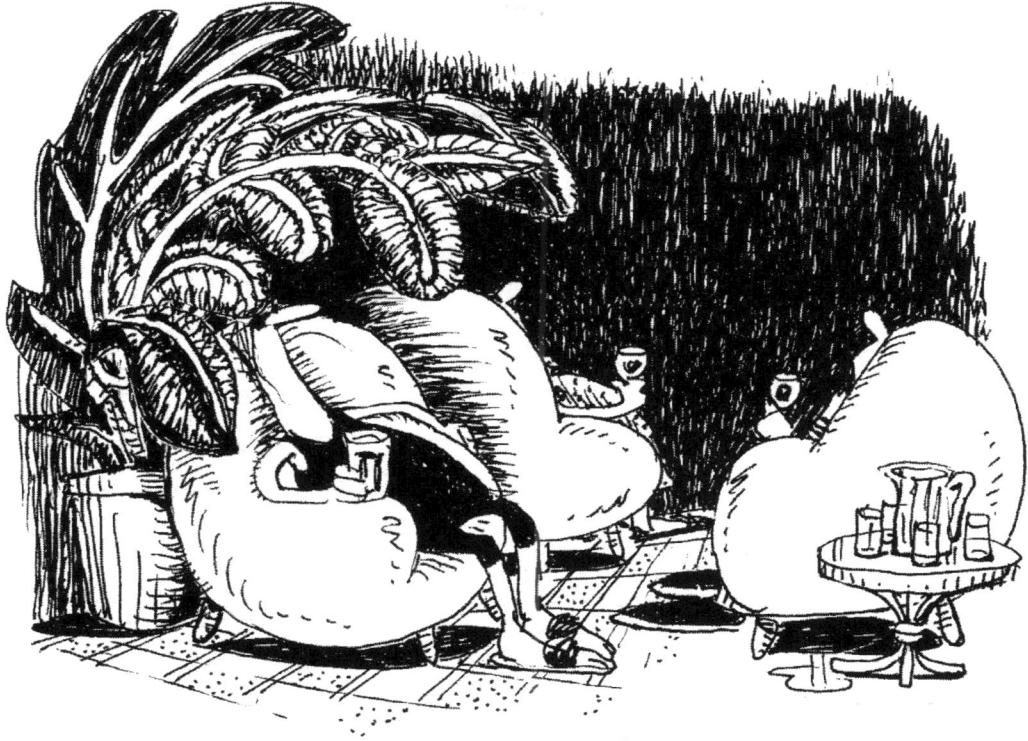

1. Good hotels

Good hotels treat their guests like royalty, and will cater to your special needs. For the chronically pained, room service is very important. So are handy ice machines. But good hotels can cost serious money.

2. Rental Apartments

A great, short-term rental apartment or small house is often better than a mediocre hotel.

In your home-away-from-home, you have privacy, lots of room and a working kitchen for drinks, ice and late-night snacks, even if you never cook an actual meal. You also have the added advantage of a living room where you and your Travel Saint can hang out when not sightseeing. Or sleeping.

It's convenient to have a place where you both have your own rooms but still live in the same space.

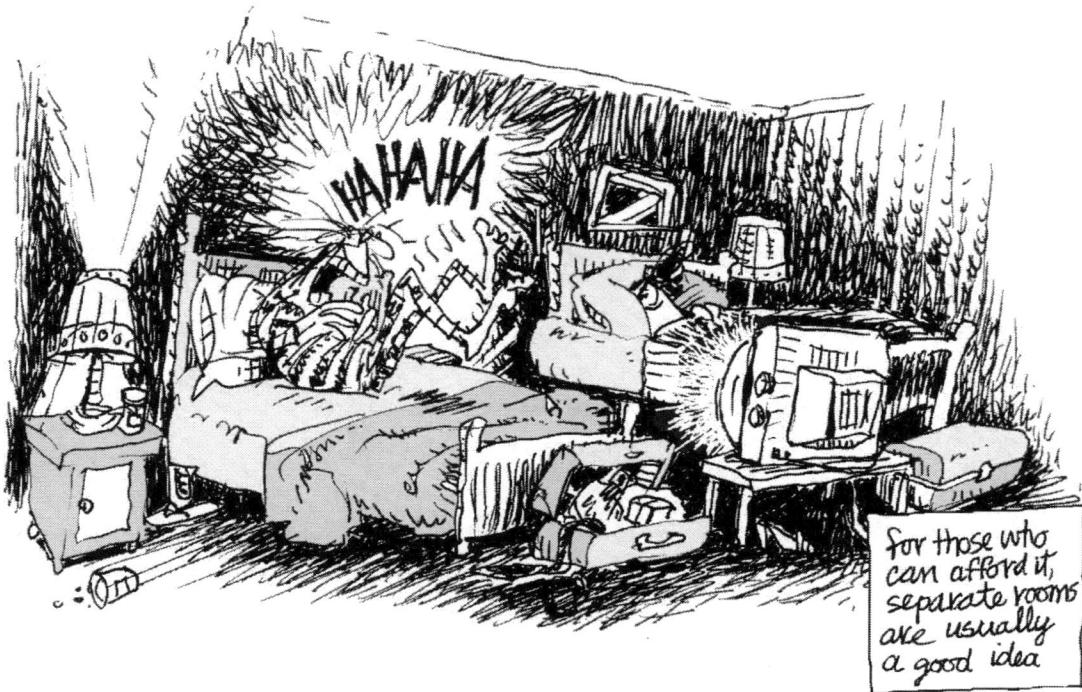

for those who can afford it, separate rooms are usually a good idea

Most two-bedroom rentals have one large master bedroom and one somewhat smaller bedroom.

Let Travel Saints have the bigger room: they deserve it, and the second bedroom, often at the back, often with fewer or smaller windows, is generally quieter, a major plus when pain necessitates lying down in the middle of the day. Just make sure both rooms have easy access to a bathroom.

Rental apartments and apartment hotels are available in a multitude of countries at various price points. Look online or ask your travel agent to look for you.

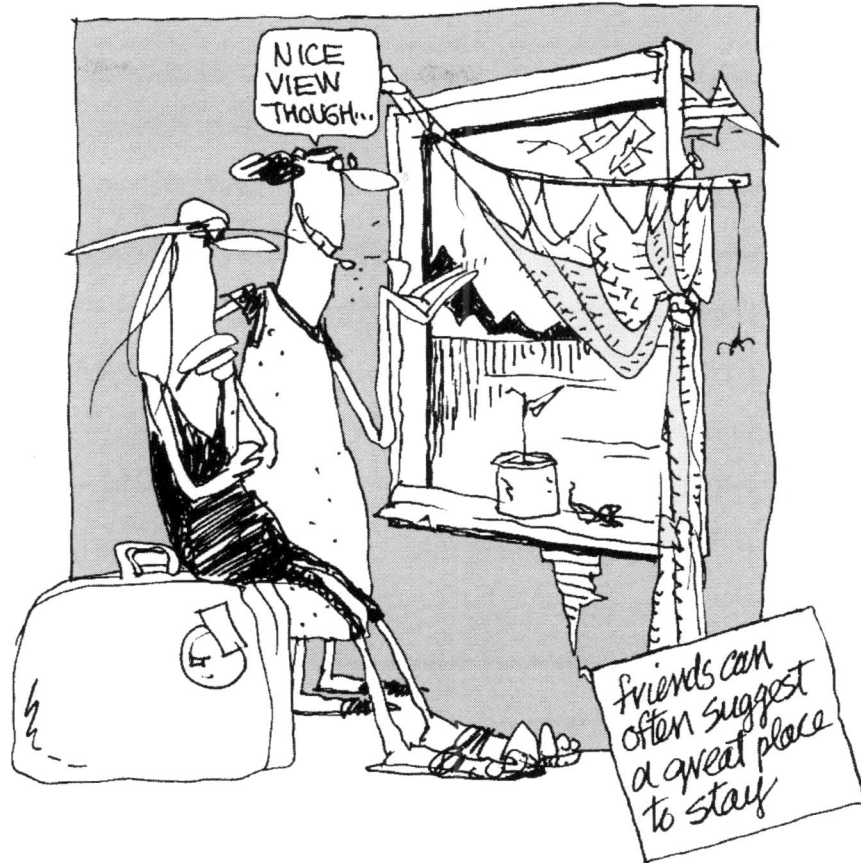

NICE VIEW THOUGH...

friends can often suggest a great place to stay

3. All-Inclusive Resorts

If you're looking for a low-stress vacation, all-inclusive resorts are perfect. Transportation, lodging, meal plans, and often tipping are included in the price and side-trips to points of interest are easily booked once you're there. All you have to do is get to the airport — once onboard the plane you can leave the rest to them. They'll meet the plane with a bus or jitney and whisk you off to the resort.

Before you book, a careful reading of the resort's website or brochure will give you a feel for the kind of people the resort is targeting. Check out the activities and amenities being offered: if you're not part of a romantic couple, it's unlikely you'll want to stay at a resort offering candlelit dinners for two and heart-shaped beds. Similarly, if you're not traveling with your own darling children, a resort geared to kiddie fun probably won't be for you. But don't worry — all-inclusive resorts are very popular. If this is the kind of stress-free vacation you'd like, there will be one that's ideal for you.

4. Cruises

Cruises are very similar to all-inclusive resorts in that they offer a complete package. For a low-stress holiday with interesting stops along the route, this is an excellent choice for people with chronic pain.

One caveat: Resorts, cruises and RV parks are all designed for people who enjoy spending time with their own kind. Most of them offer various get-togethers, activities and events where guests can meet and mingle. But if you want to meet people from different cultures and experience the world on a more intimate level with locals, the all-inclusive, somewhat exclusive holiday might not be your best choice.

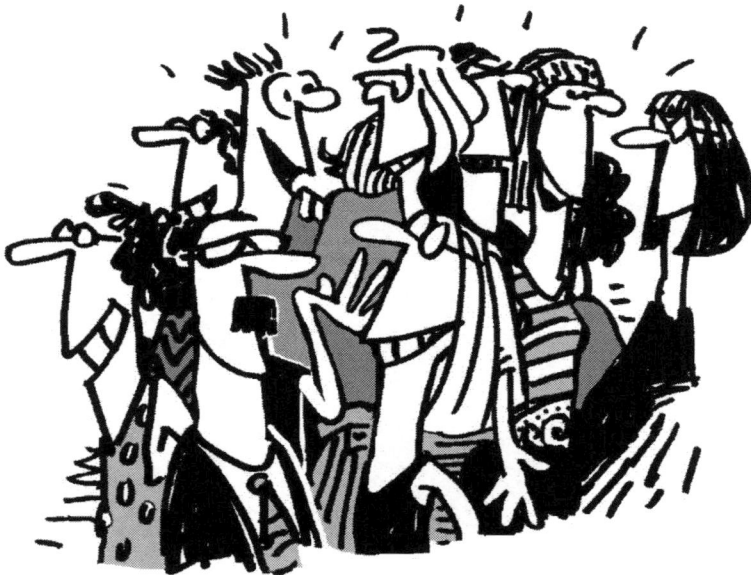

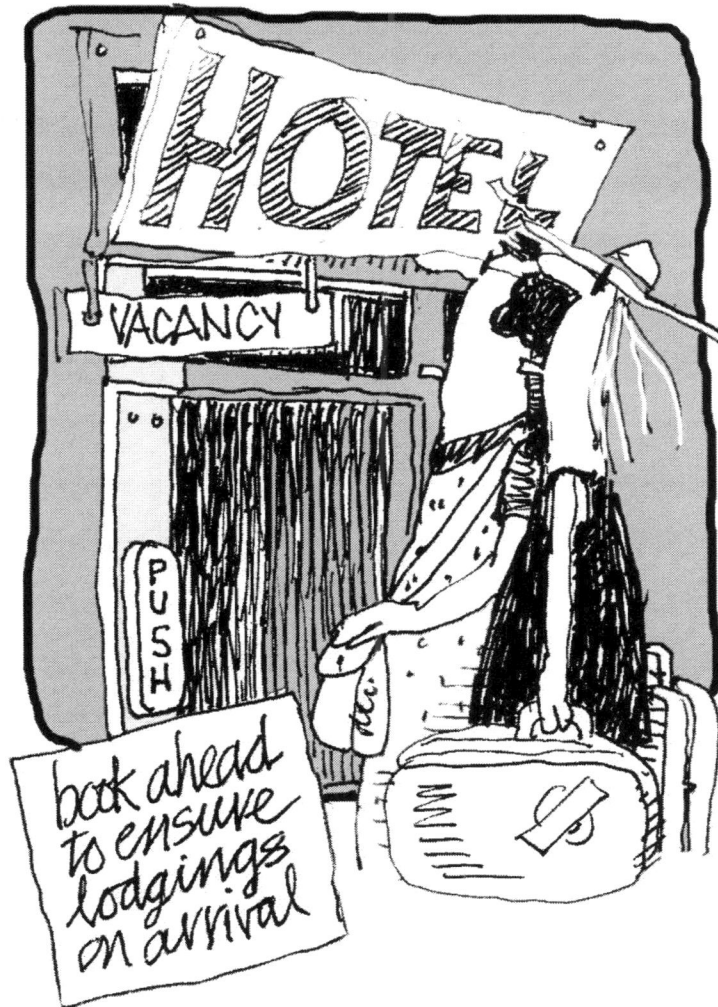

My Not So Faves

1. Bed & Breakfasts

Perhaps I'm alone in feeling the bed & breakfast experience should be avoided like the plague. But seriously, for those of us who occasionally need to spend the day in bed, why would we choose a place where we're expected to leave after breakfast? And speaking of breakfast, you're supposed to eat the delicious, homemade meal your hosts got up at some ungodly hour to prepare. I'm as sociable as the next person, but I'm uber cranky at breakfast. Cramming down coffee, orange juice and a croissant while still half asleep and before the pain meds kick in is no time for amusing banter.

However, if you're a chatty type who wants to get to know local folks, a B&B could be just right for you.

2. Camping

Some people who suffer from chronic pain camp in spite of it. Most don't.

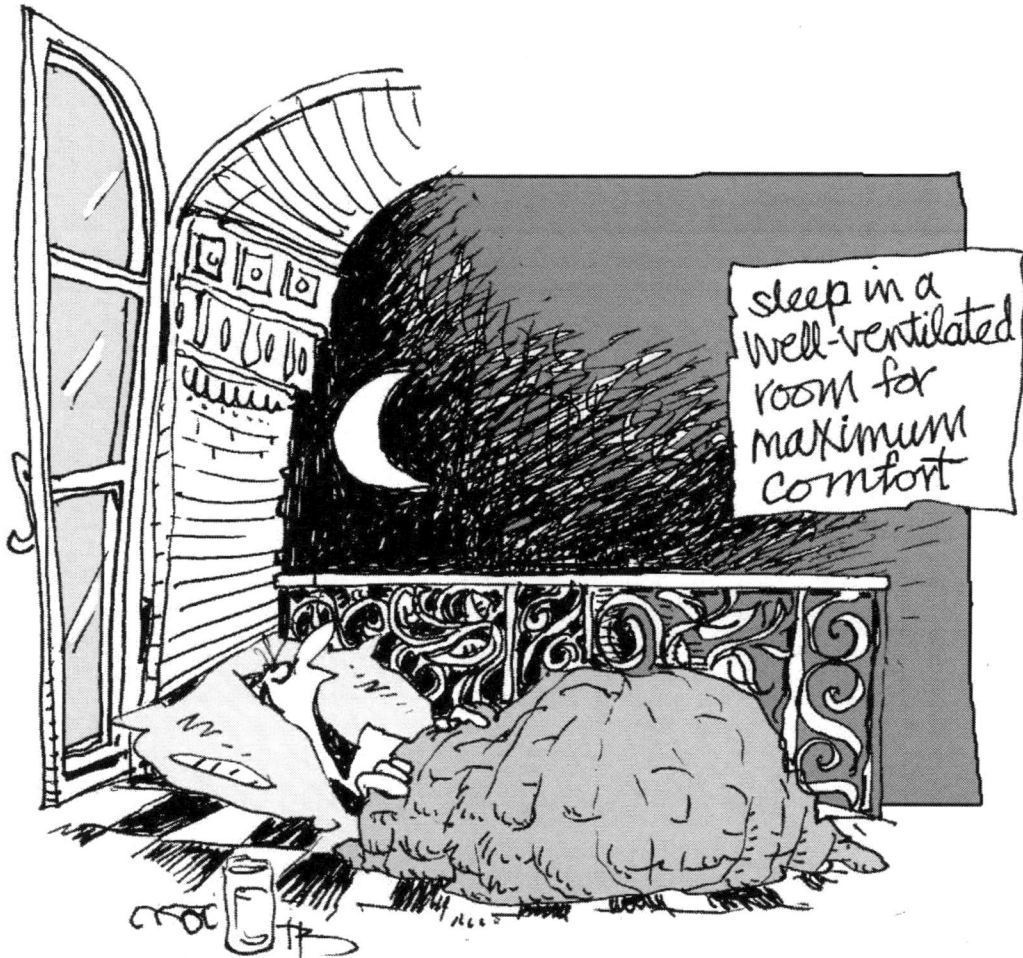

LOCATION, LOCATION, LOCATION!

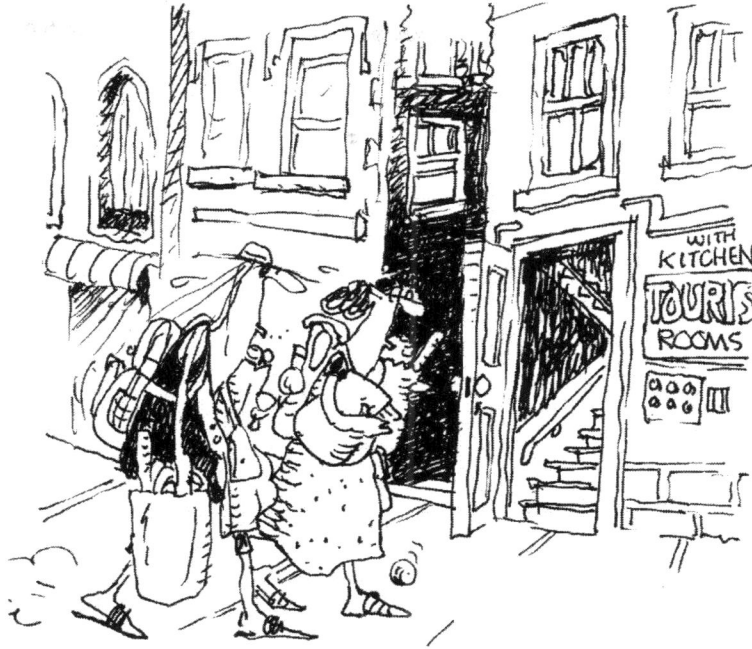

If you're sensitive to noise you probably don't want to stay on the main drag, but do make sure that wherever you stay is located close to, or in the heart of, the area where you'll want to spend most of your time. When your energy is limited by chronic pain, even half an hour getting to and from the high spots is annoying. And there are times when the pain makes it urgent that you get back to your digs quickly.

Lying in the back of a taxi, groaning, is not a great way to spend your holiday.

Soon after you arrive, try to find a decent restaurant very near your place that has takeout for those days when you're simply not up to cooking or going out to eat. When you're in too much pain to move, your companion can buy something without hunting all over town or either of you going hungry. Also make note of the closest bakery or deli for the same reason.

Whether you choose a hotel, an apartment or a B&B, research carefully and book well ahead of your trip. Thanks to the Internet, you can leave very little to chance. Photos will tell you if it's the kind of place you'd want to stay, but pay attention to decor! A ratty sofa speaks volumes about general upkeep.

Google Maps will show you how close it is to the sights you want to visit. Travelers often try to cram as many places as possible into their vacation, booking new accommodations in each center. For people with chronic pain, it's much easier to establish a home base, unpack and stay in one spot for the entire time you're away. You can relax in your home base, really get to know the area you've chosen and take day trips from there.

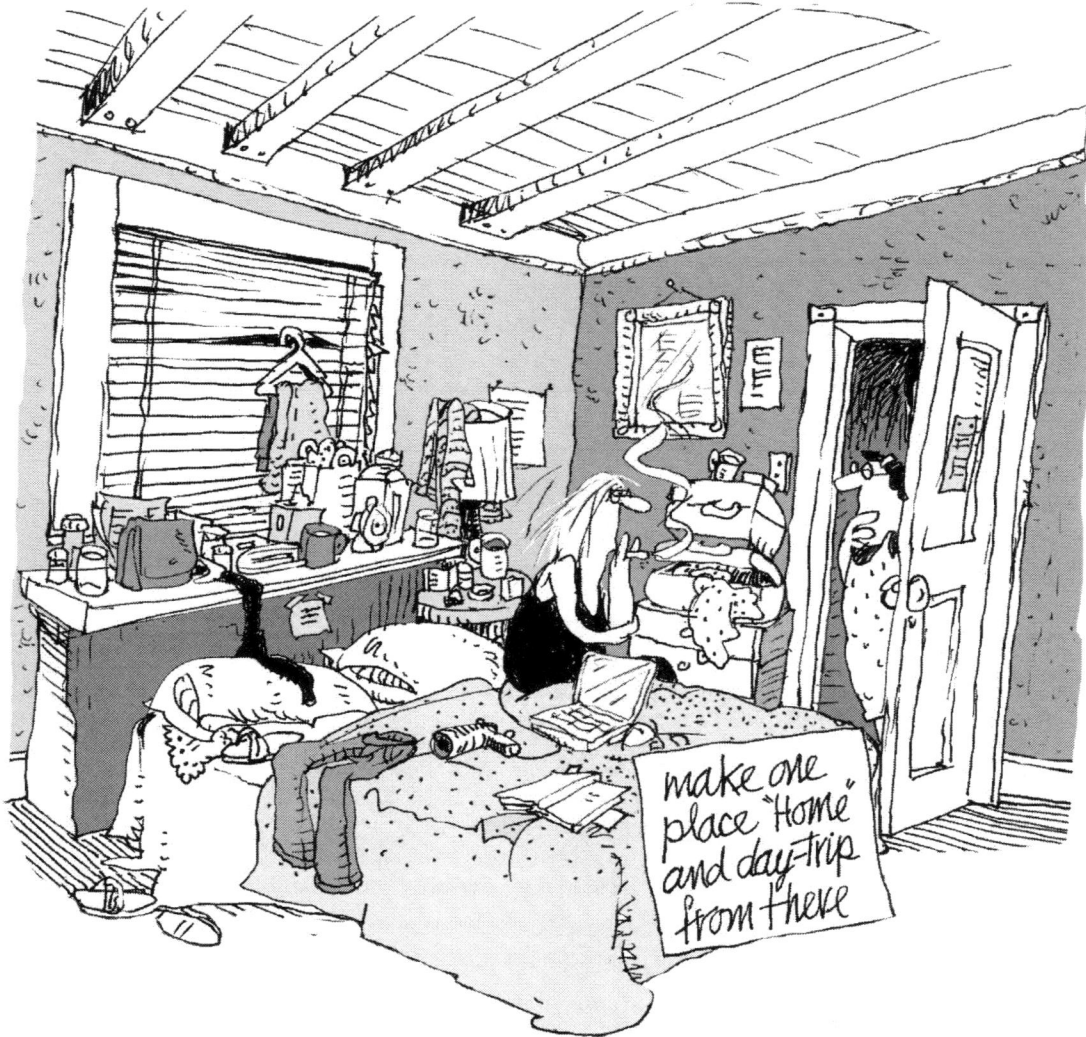

One caveat: make sure your accommodation is on the ground floor or there's an elevator. You don't want to be hauling yourself or your heavy suitcases up six floors. And you can't expect the Travel Saint to do it for you.

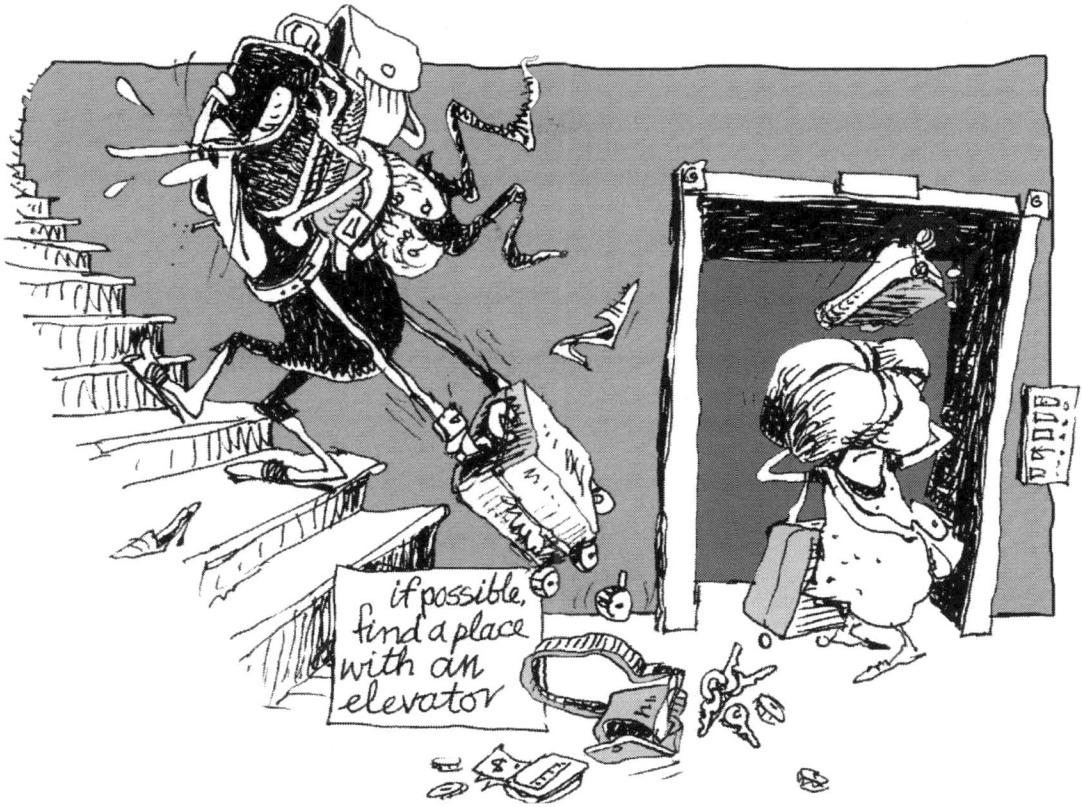

if possible,
find a place
with an
elevator

There are limits, even for saints

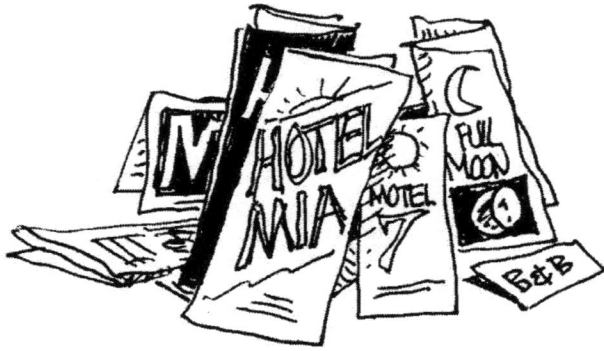

Chapter 6
SHARING

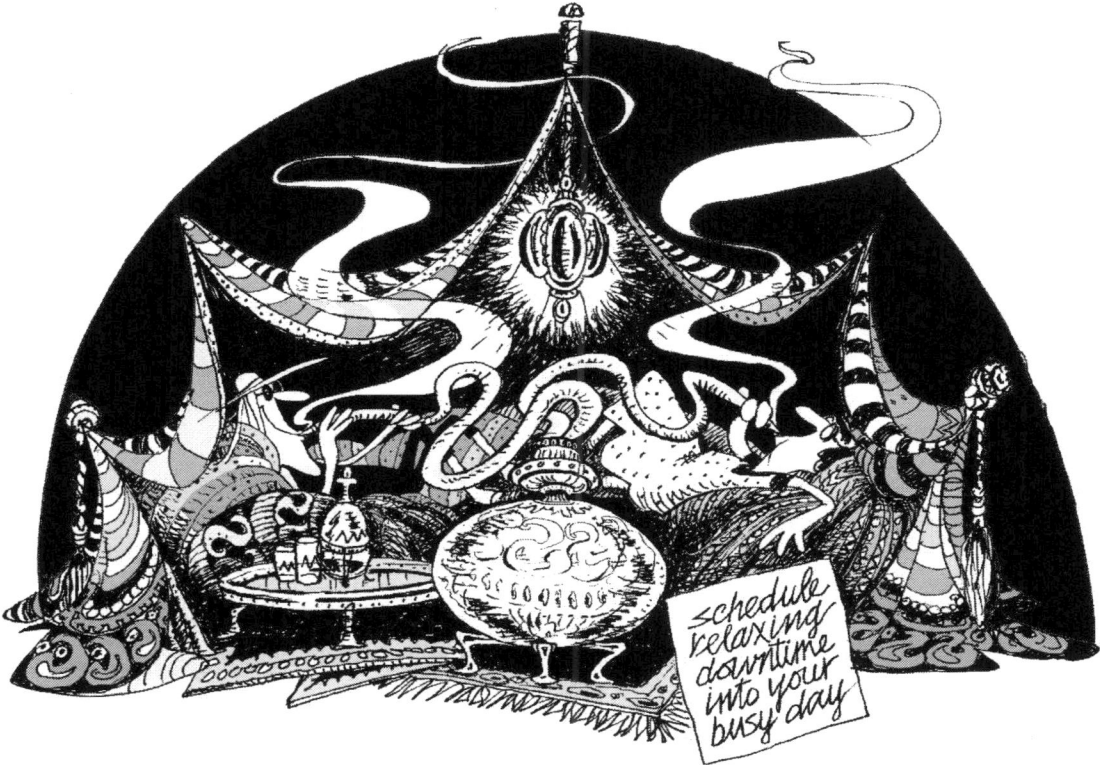

schedule relaxing downtime into your busy day

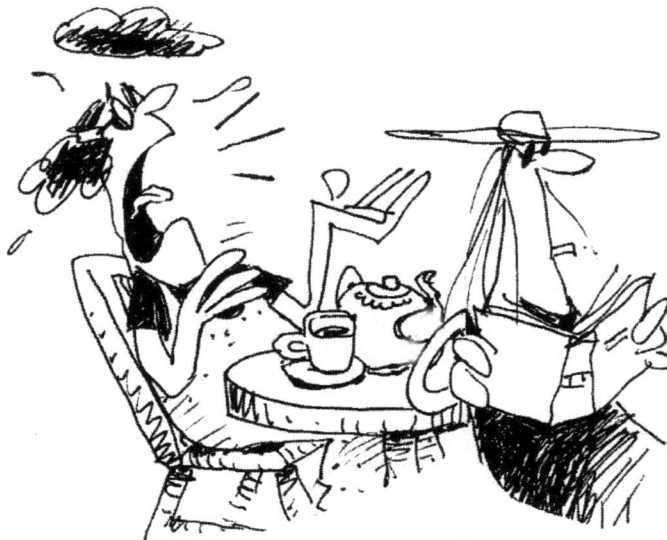

*Have an honest conversation with your potential roommate
before booking shared accommodation*

Sharing travel and accommodation with someone other than your life partner can be stressful at times. Even if you're traveling with a best friend, someone you've known for years, things will come up when you're spending day and night together, things you never knew about each other . . . and sometimes things you'd rather not know.

You'll also make wonderful discoveries—he or she hasn't been your friend for nothing. But no matter who your travel partner is, the best rule of thumb is honesty. If you're very honest about what your needs will be and what your infirmity may possibly or absolutely require, your travel pal will feel more comfortable telling you his or her particular needs and expectations.

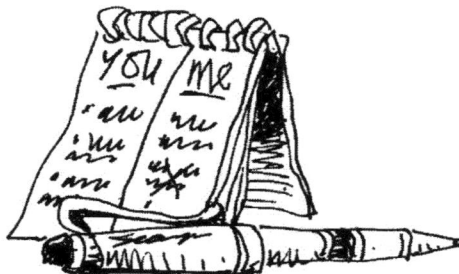

This conversation should take place once you've decided you'd like to travel together but before you've actually booked passage. It's only reasonable to let potential travel partners off the hook if they'd rather not contend with your chronic pain. If you're great friends, your health problems won't come as a complete surprise. But very few people who don't either suffer from chronic pain themselves, or live with someone who does, really understand the intricacies of dealing with chronic pain on a daily basis. It's up to you to disclose as much as you think is fair.

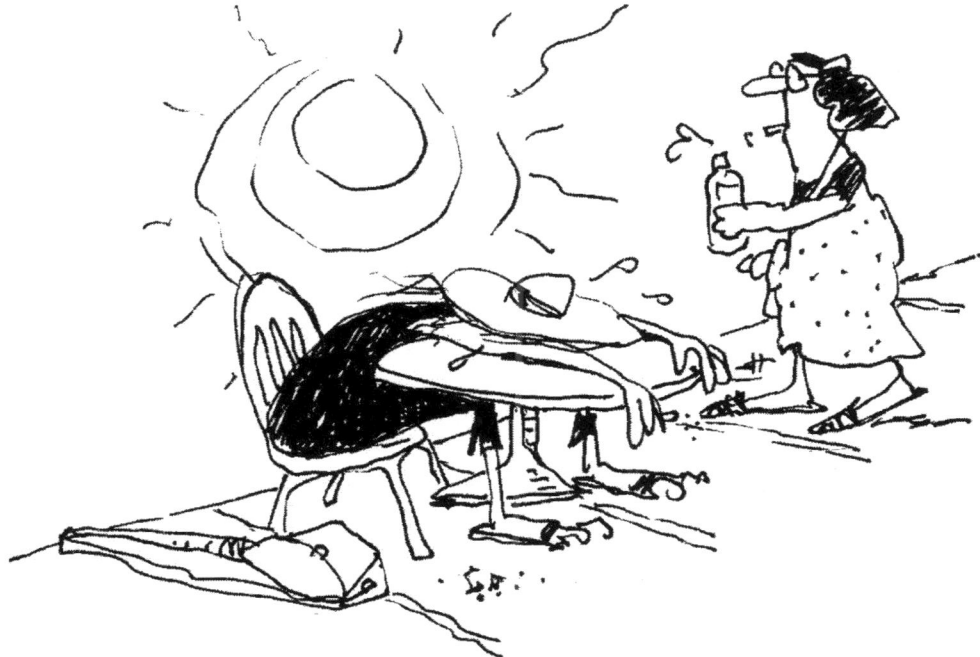

"What is fair?" you ask.

Think about what your travel partner needs to know that he or she might not know. Pain imposes some limitations on what or how much you're able to do: how far you can walk, how fast you can walk, how many places you can see in a day will all be limited, to a certain extent, by your health. If there will be days (or hours) when you need to lie down, if there will be times you'll need to take major drugs, if there might be trips to a doctor or emergency department, your travel partner should know these things.

But it's also important for the other to know that you are a strong, self-sufficient, honest and uncomplaining partner. You're not looking for a Travel Nurse, just a partner who understands your limitations.

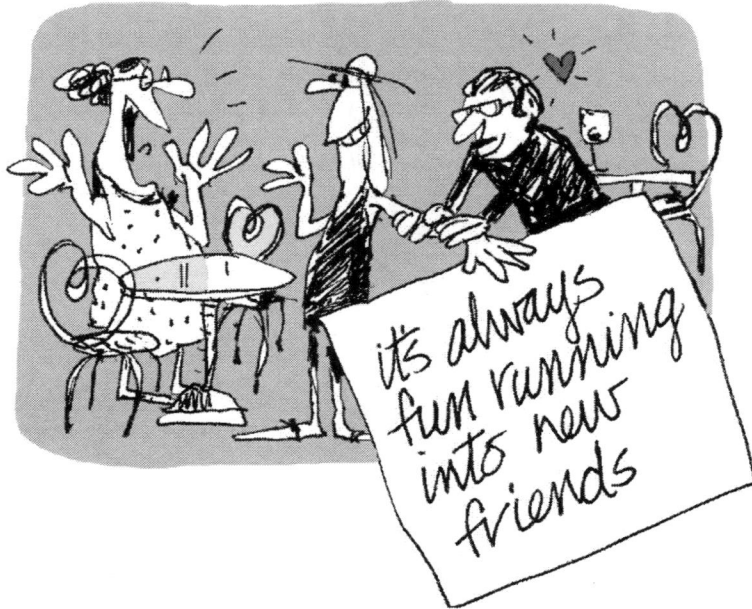

If your pain actually requires a little help now and then, be specific about what kind of help you'd like. No one can read your mind, but most people are very willing to help a friend when they know what's needed.

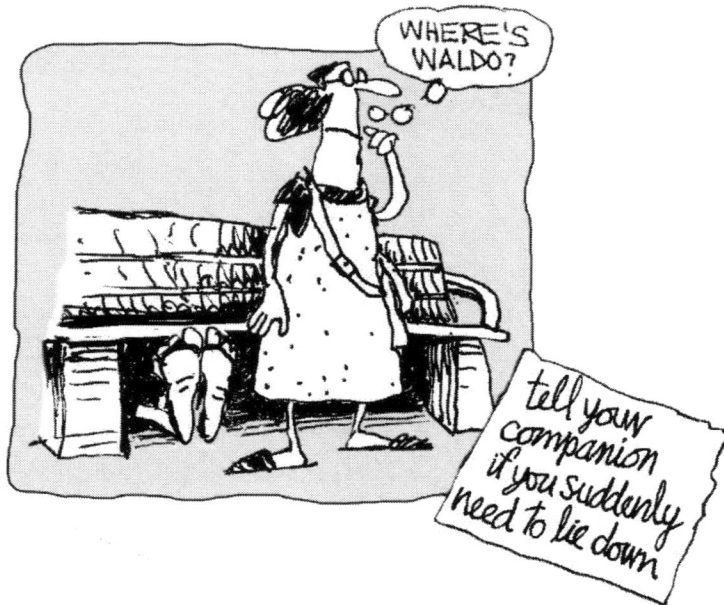

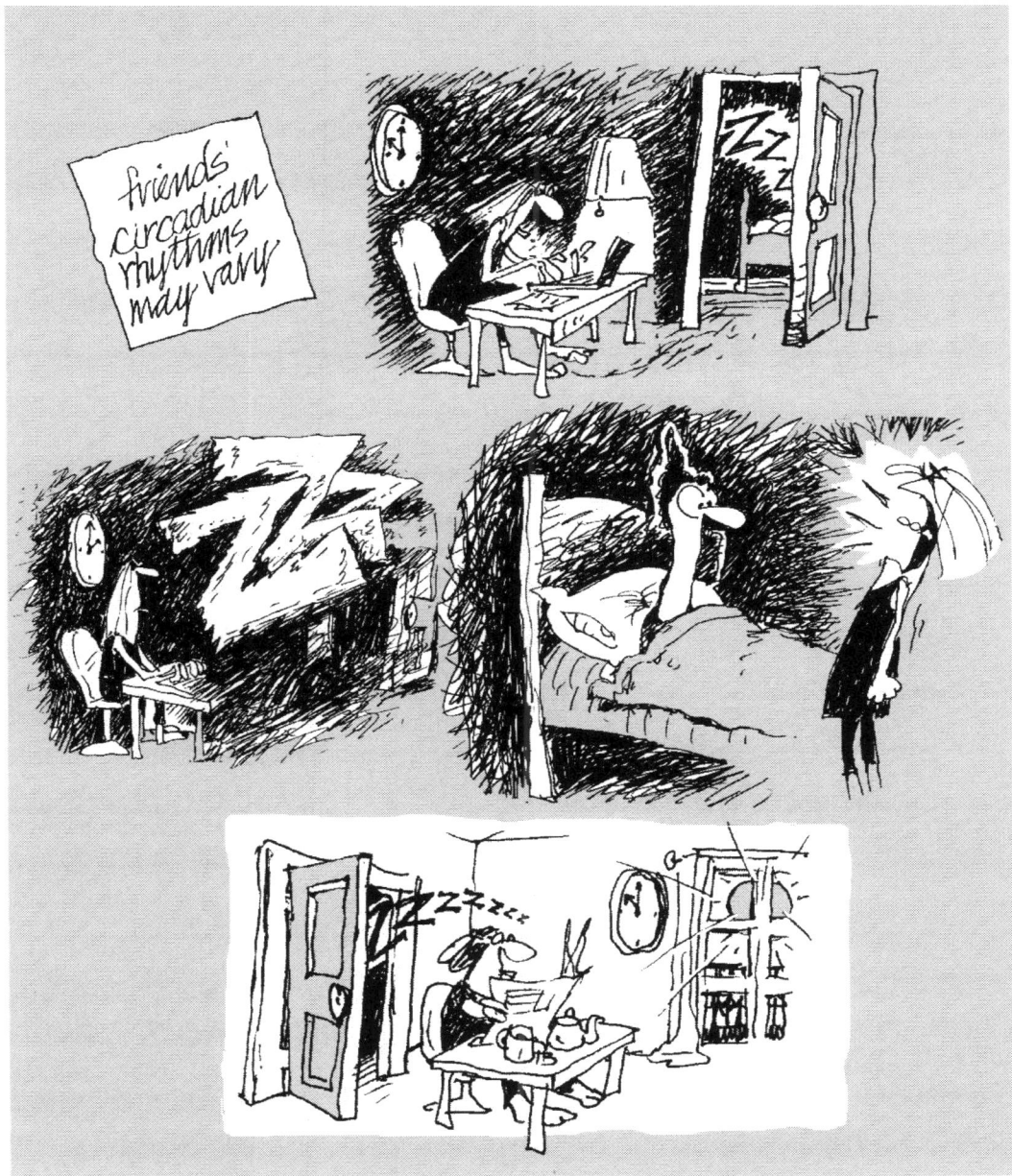

People with chronic pain are always trying to find a balance between being non-complaining, soldiering on, trying to get above the pain on the one hand, and yet being honest with others when the pain is so great that they must give in to it. More than anything, chronic pain makes us a little unreliable—no one knows when we'll be unable to go on. But if your travel partners are aware of all this ahead of time (and if they're good friends, they probably already know most of it), you'll be comfortable traveling together.

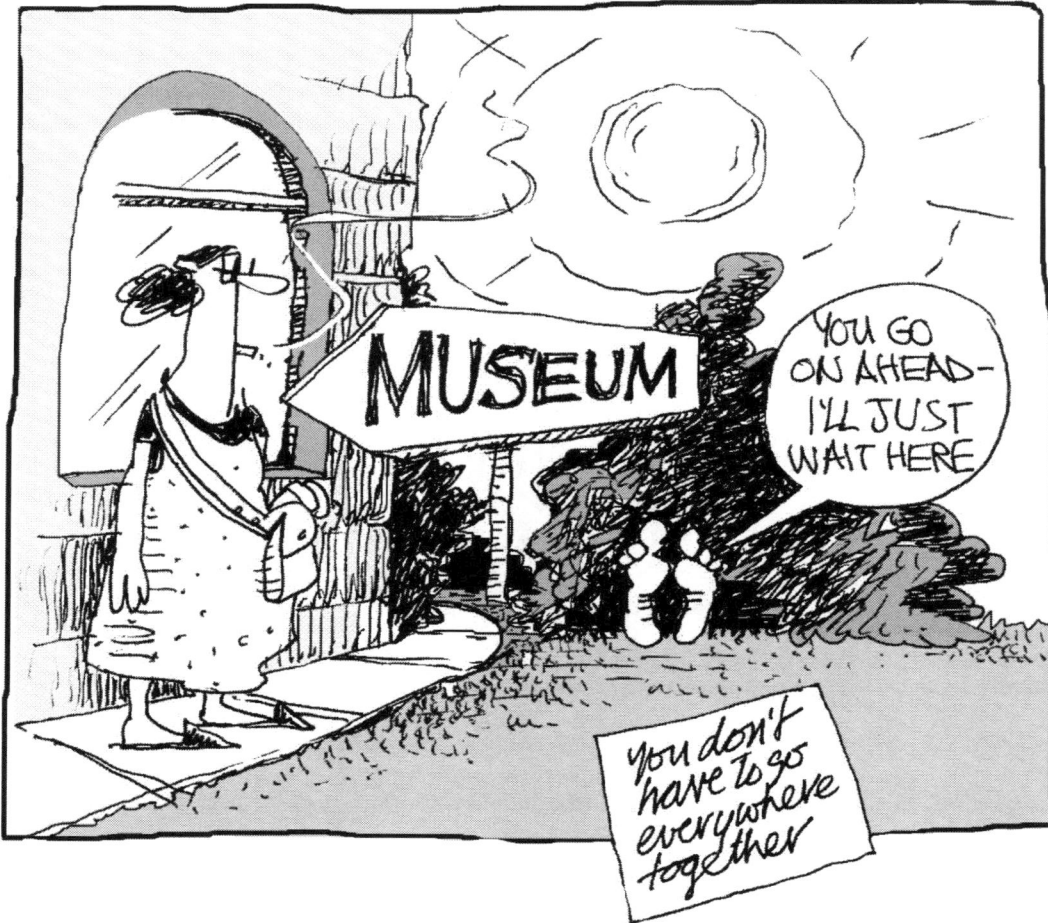

I refer to my usual travel partner as the Travel Saint because she is so good with me when I'm incapacitated. She's steered me through Paris crowds, hailed impossible-to-hail taxis in Athens, and brought me food pretty well everywhere we've been. Not that this happens all the time, or even every day, but the times I've overdone it, I would have been in dire straits if it weren't for her selfless understanding and capability. So pick your travel partner with some care.

Of course, we do things for each other; at times, I'm probably her Travel Saint too. And that's all to the good — it balances things out.

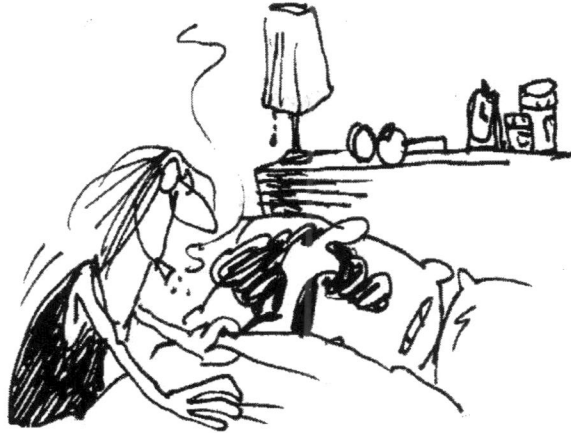

You may be sharing almost everything, but a little time away from each other is good—just like in a marriage, time spent apart brings conversational interest back to your meals or outings. If you're not feeling up to traipsing around one day, spend the time in your hotel getting better while your partner takes in a sight you don't absolutely need to see.

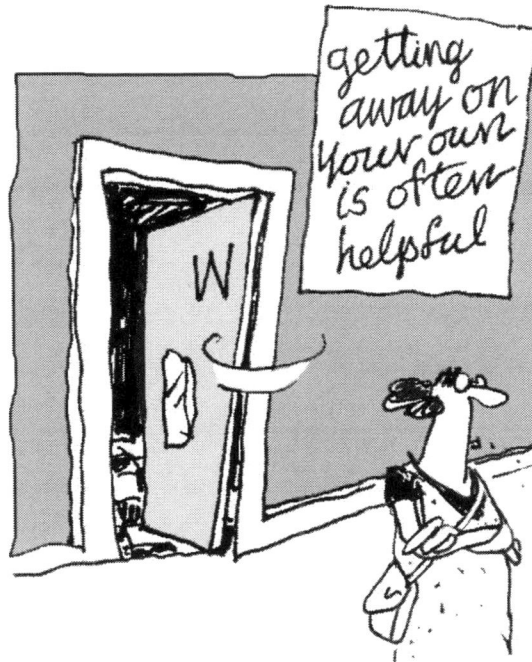

getting away on your own is often helpful

Or if you're anxious to see a particular site and your partner isn't that interested, split up for a while and go your separate ways. You'll have lots to show and tell when you meet up again.

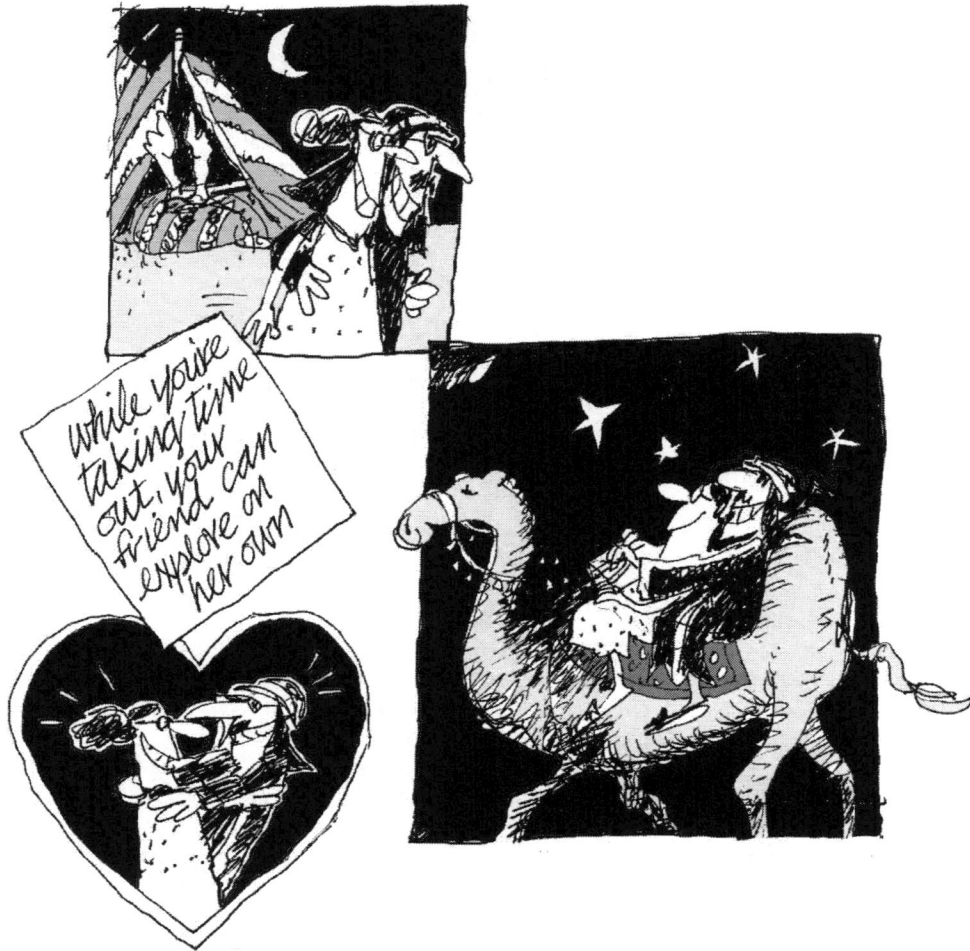

while you're taking time out, your friend can explore on her own

Sharing an apartment or hotel room is like most things in life: everything works better with manners, which means thinking about your companion.

When you keep your stuff tucked away in your room—or part of the room—and don't leave dirty dishes, clothes, or purchases lying around willy-nilly, you're showing consideration. It may not be the way you live at home, but it's really important when sharing.

Saying please and thank you ensures the Travel Saint doesn't feel taken for granted. And being aware of the other's needs—everyone can use a little help now and then—makes daily life a pleasure, not a burden.

If your travel pal is looking after you a bit when you're under the weather, doing something nice in return is appreciated. It's definitely not a tit-for-tat gesture, but by thinking of your friend and bringing back flowers for the apartment or croissants fresh from your early morning walk, you're saying thank you. Small niceties go a long way toward making your Saint feel appreciated.

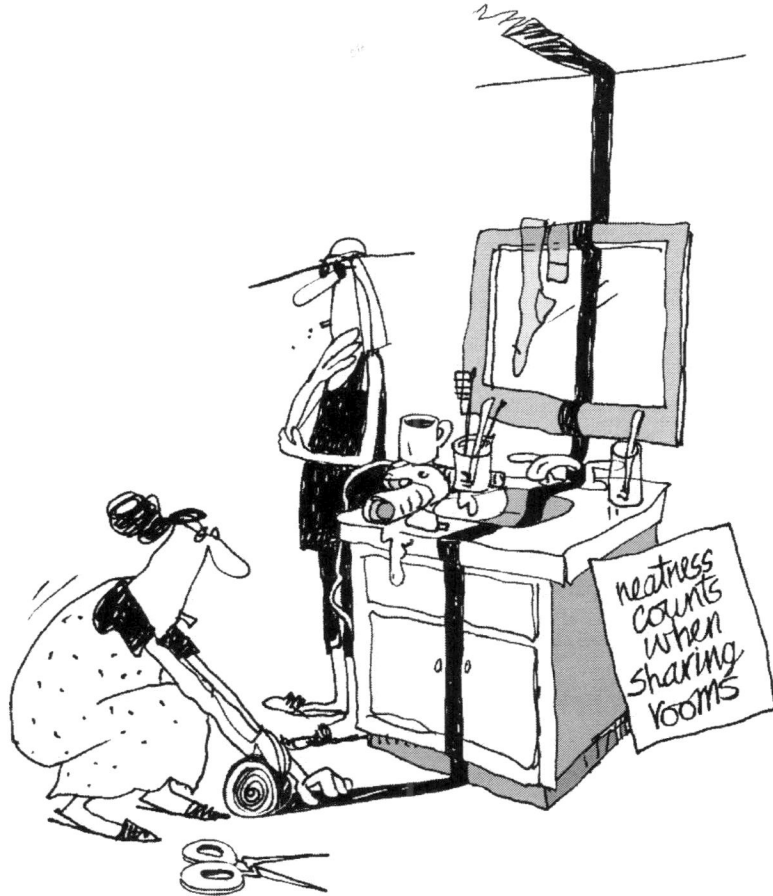

Sometimes, hurt feelings happen. Just the fact that neither of you is used to spending so much time together almost ensures that at some point in the trip, one of you will say or do something that irritates the other. Pretending it hasn't happened is not usually a good idea. Things fester. The sooner you can talk about this, apologize if necessary and laugh about it, the more quickly it'll be forgotten and the two of you can move on to another enjoyable day.

Above all, sharing a trip should be fun. You'll have great memories of the time you spent together and will laugh about the details with each other for the rest of your lives.

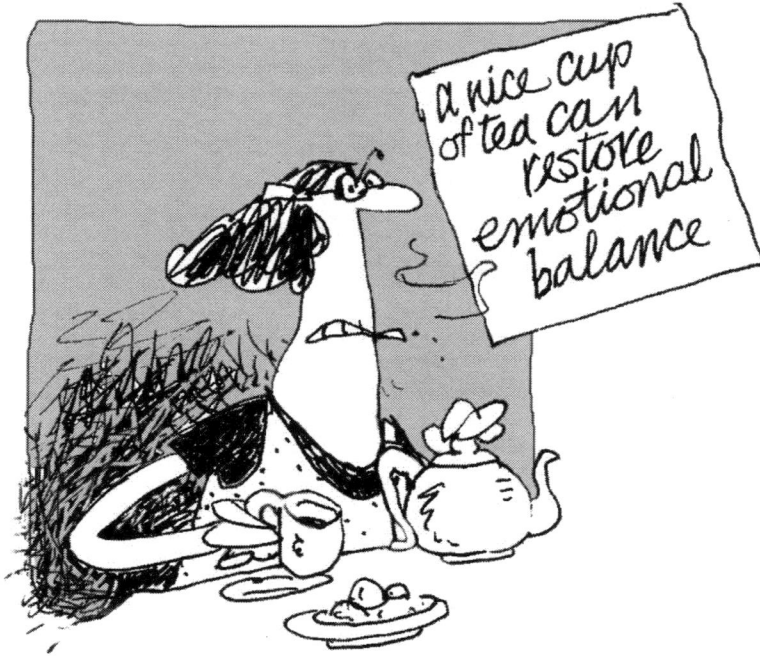

Chapter 7
SIGHTSEEING

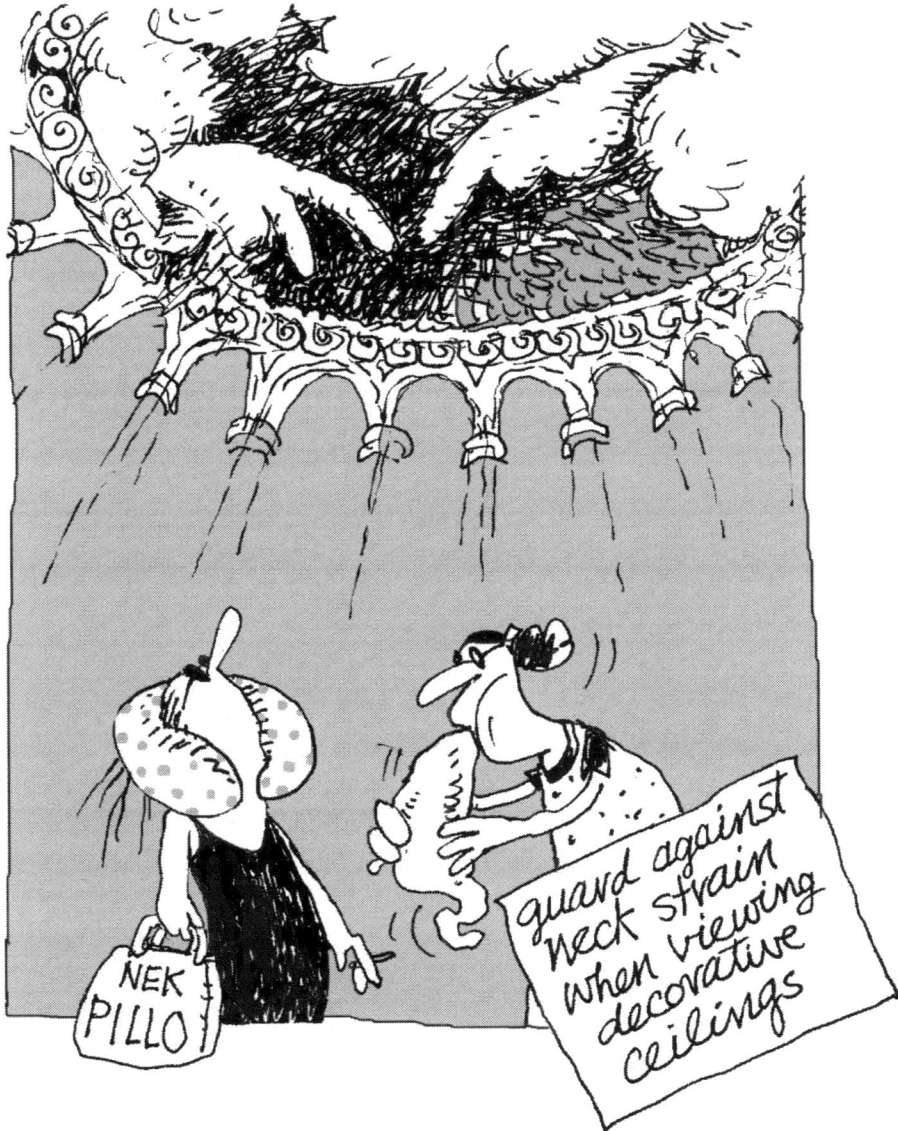

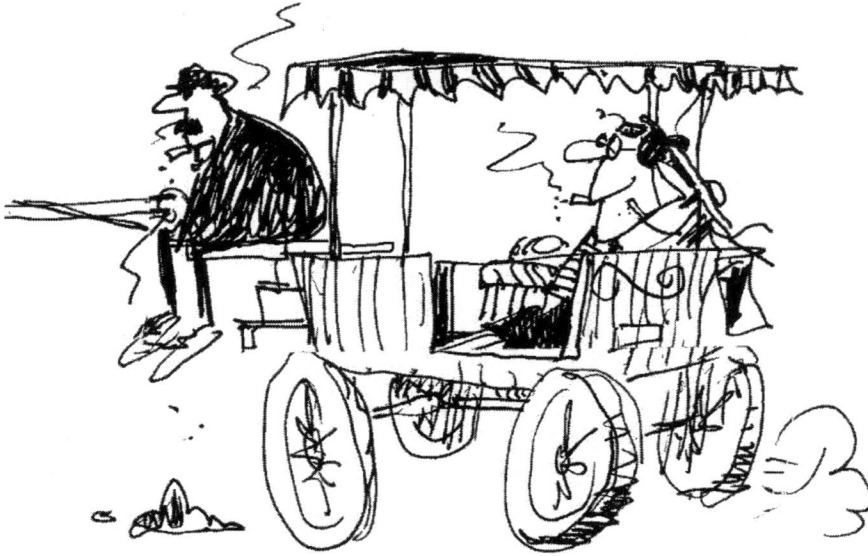

An ability to accept change can lead to a far richer life

Before You Leave Home

Plan, plan, plan! Wherever your chosen destination lies, you'll find sights (and sites) to see. You and your Travel Saint will both want to explore some things while perhaps only one of you will have much interest in other places.

The best thing to do is to gather as much information as you can on the area before you leave home, and list the places you both absolutely MUST see, which ones you both have some interest in and which spots only one of you wants to visit.

Then get hold of an area map. Google Maps are terrific—print one out beforehand if you don't think you'll be able to find a map at the local tourist board (and often the tourist maps are inadequate). Use a felt pen to mark the places with numbers or stars, note which ones are close together and might be seen at the same time. Check if there's a shopping area you want to visit close to the site. Then lay out a calendar and plan your attack.

But remember, while your companion may be able to take in several sites at once, you may not. Personally, I find one major site a day the most I can do. You know your own tolerance for walking, gazing, taking in information. Work to that.

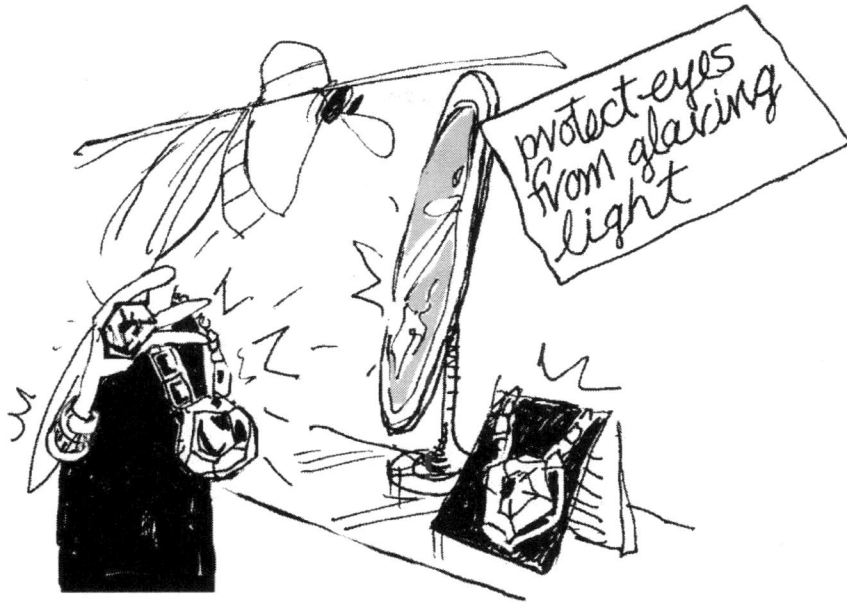

You're There!

Be sure to take supplies you might need when away from your home base for a long stretch: medication for the day, water, sunglasses, extra sweater or jacket, folding cane if the terrain will be rough. But remember, you'll have to carry this stuff all day, so pack as lightly as possible.

Some people feel safer wearing a money belt for their cash and passport. But these days, when bank machines and credit cards are the norm, it's no longer necessary to carry large amounts of cash or travelers' checks, and many people feel quite safe keeping their money in a front pocket or closely held purse. Your hotel will likely allow you to use its safe for your passport (if you haven't already had to surrender it at the desk). Using common sense is your best safety plan, just as it is at home.

Before starting out on your own, consider taking a comfortable, air-conditioned, guided tour bus for an hour or two. It's a great way to get a feel for what and where you'd like to visit. If you prefer a more leisurely pace, a horse-drawn carriage or rickshaw tour is fun: they usually pass by all the major spots, give you a little history and explain what you'll see at each site. And, very importantly, you'll get a good idea of the distances involved in getting there. Some places will be close enough to your hotel to walk to; others will be farther away.

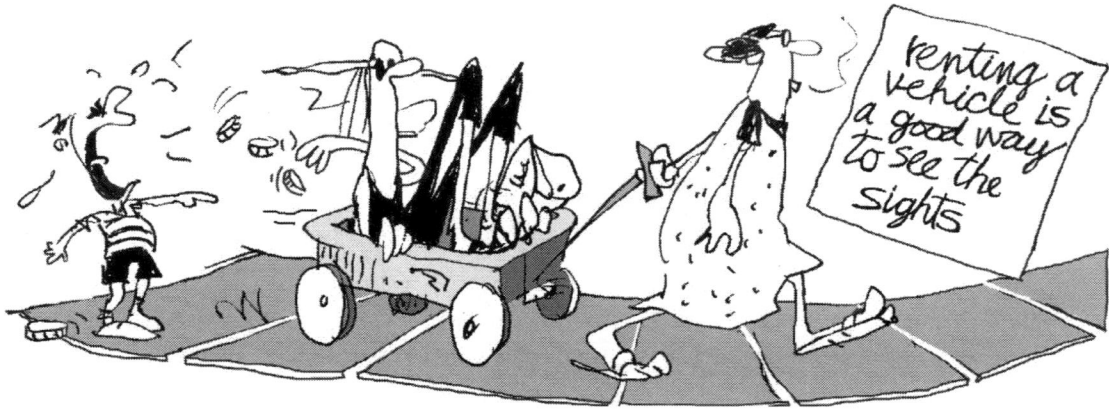

Think creatively. What are your particular interests? Maybe you want to see the factory where they make that wonderful earthenware. Maybe your companion wants to visit a local sawmill. Most factories have tours; phone and find out. If one of you visits a place the other doesn't particularly want to see, it will give you a little time away from each other and you'll both have interesting tales to tell later.

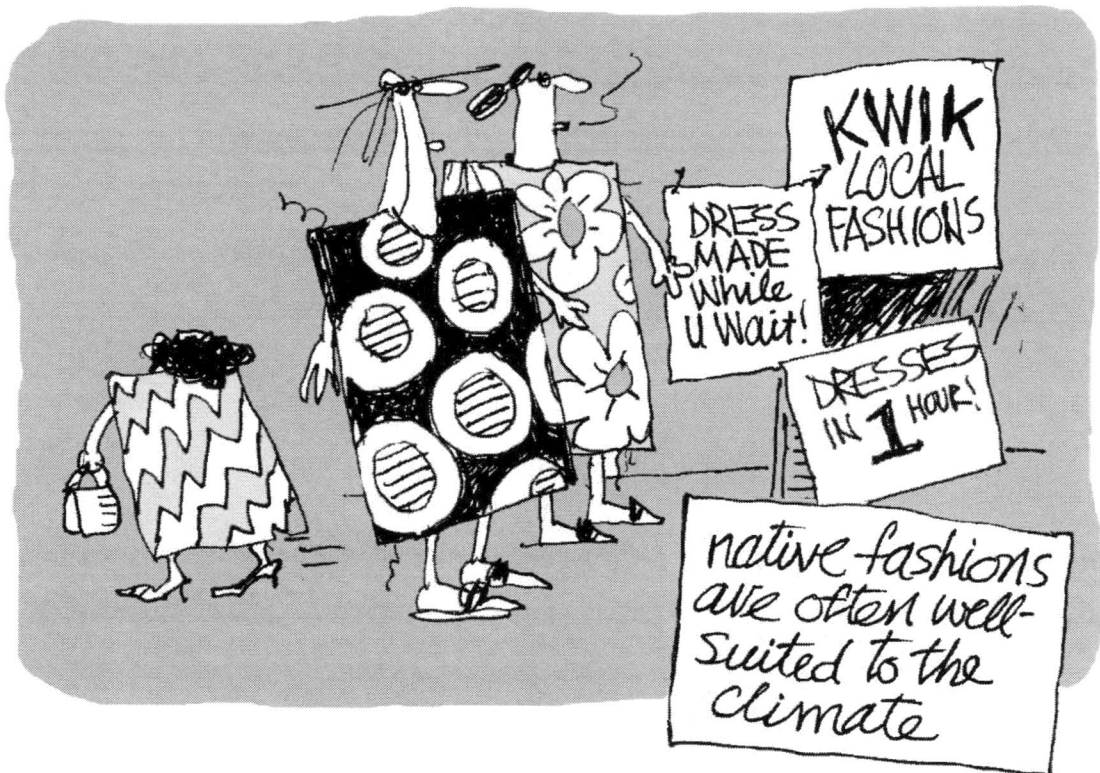

Perhaps the most important thing to remember while sightseeing is to allow enough time at each place. Small time outs (in a café or on a bench in the shade) can make it possible for you to last much longer than if you just try to press on without resting.

Quite often major places of interest are a fair distance from each other and require either driving (rental car), cabbing or public transit. Be sure to include traveling time in your calculations.

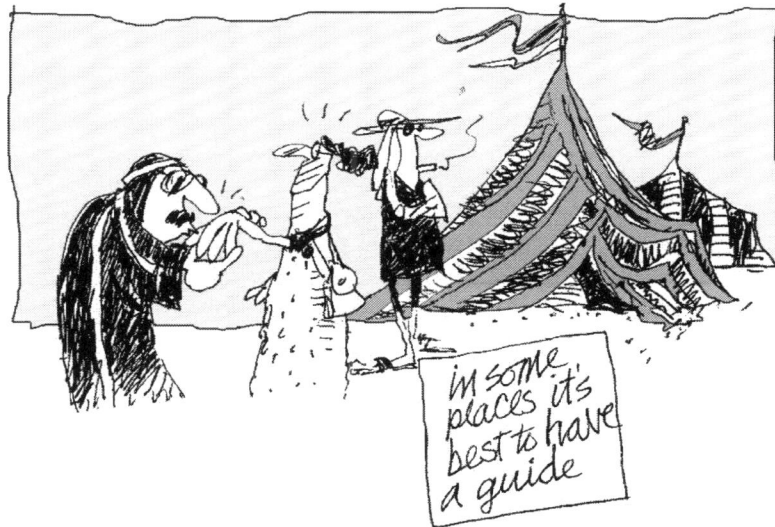

in some places it's best to have a guide

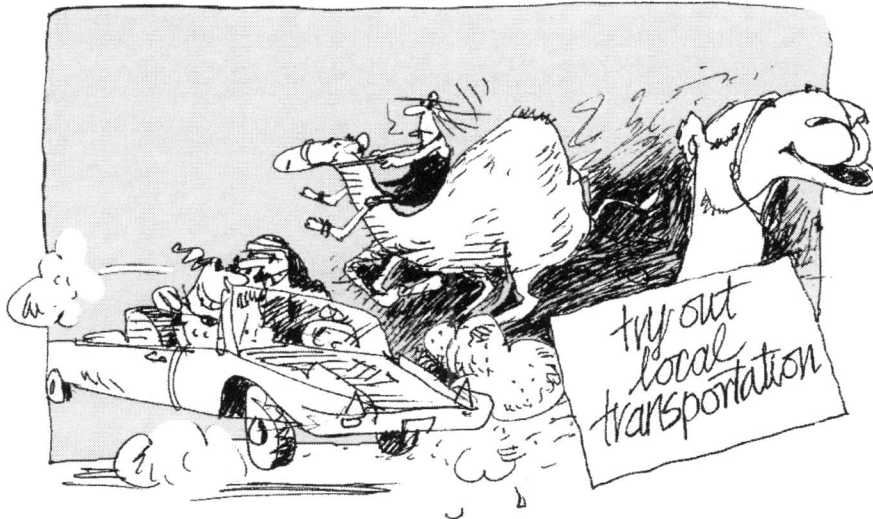

try out local transportation

Some of the sites you thought you wanted to see might not look as interesting as you expected, and you can cross them off your list. Other spots you'd never considered will be so enticing you'll add them to your agenda.

Use the Internet. If you don't have online access where you're staying, almost every city, town and even village has Internet cafés — you can find out what's open, and when. Check out whether you can buy tickets in advance, which days are discounted or, sometimes, free. Look at online pictures or photos in your guidebook to assess whether there's shade or indoor shelter, such as a cafeteria or restaurant, if that's important to you.

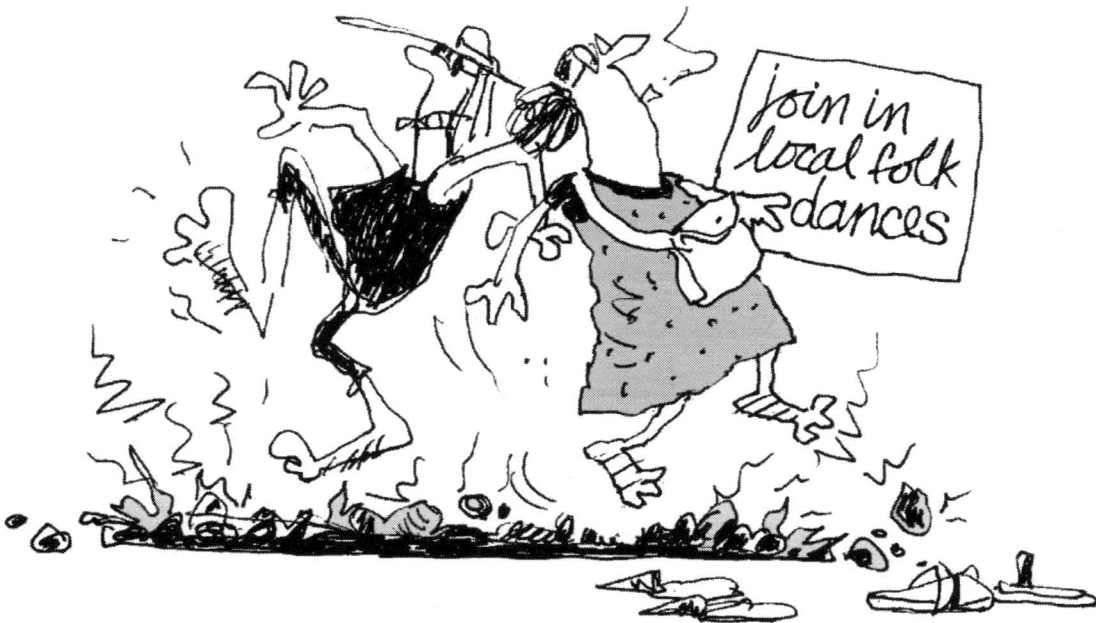

Smart phones have apps that cover most of these needs and are much lighter than books. They also have decent built-in cameras. A cell phone is handy if you and your companion become separated, but remember to check with your provider (or get a SIM card) before you leave home to avoid high roaming rates for calls and data. A folding shopping bag tucked into a purse often comes in handy. You never know what treasures you'll come across!

When mobility is an issue, look for elevators. Consider when the busiest times might be and try to go at off-peak hours to avoid long line-ups.

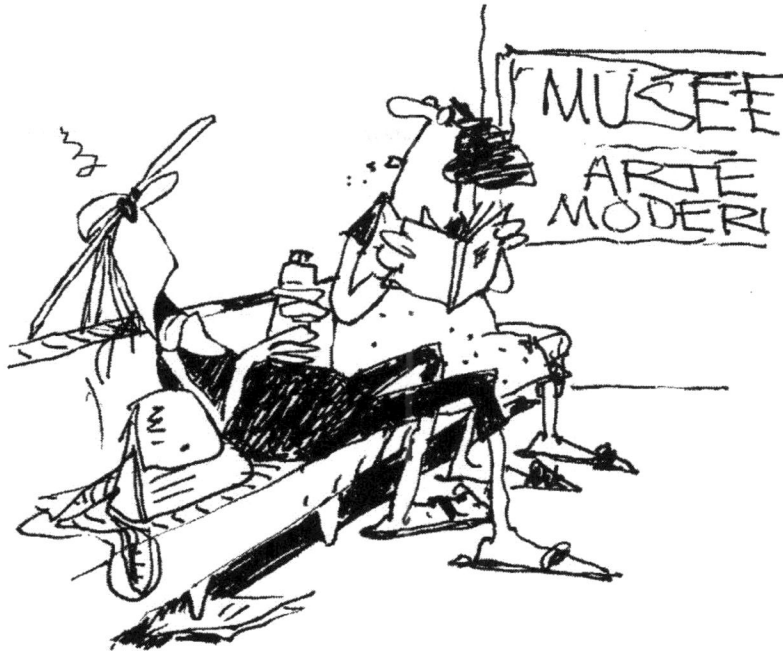

Often a person with chronic pain needs to rest in a reasonably comfortable place to regain energy. Your companion could carry on sightseeing while you sit with a cool drink and read your book or people-watch.

When sightseeing with your companion, try to share some of the things you'll need. If you're carrying guidebooks, maps or phrasebooks around with you, share the load.

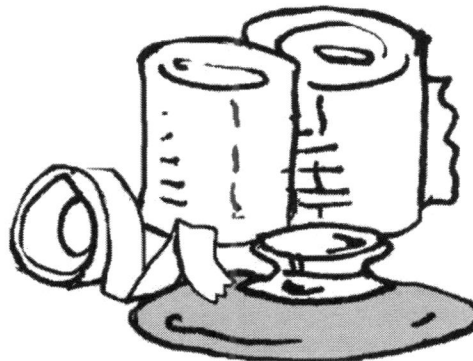

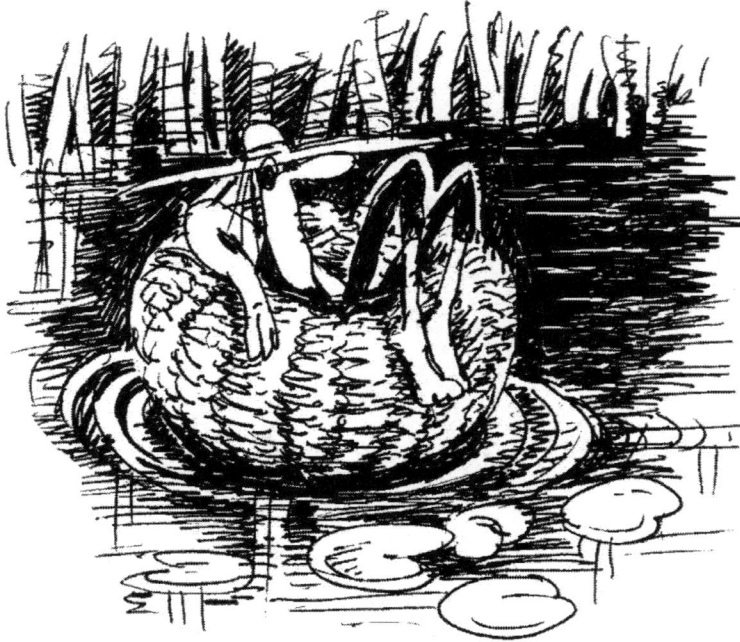

In spite of your best-laid plans, some days you're just not up to sightseeing at all. While you rest and recuperate, your companion could take in a few of the sights you're not committed to visiting. And the two of you can adjust your schedule to accommodate something you both want to see on another day. Don't worry if you can't manage to check off absolutely everything on your agenda. Enjoying the places you do see is much more important.

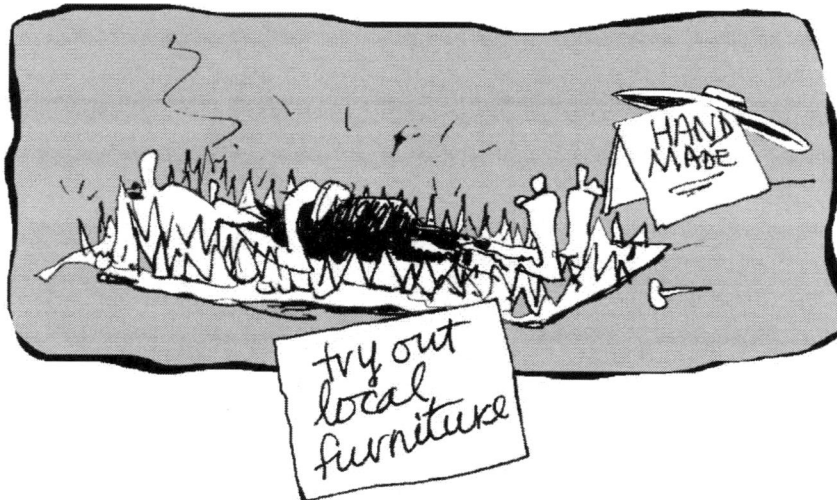

Visit the gift shop in a museum, church or gallery. You'll probably find wonderful, site-specific items to take back to your friends at home. Visit the café, if there is one. It might have special local treats. Buy postcards, take pictures, enjoy the outing. And if the neighborhood where the gallery, monument, cathedral, etc. is located looks interesting, take the time to wander around. Smaller, local galleries are often situated close to a major gallery but not indicated on tourist maps. Quaint outdoor restaurants might be just around the corner from a museum.

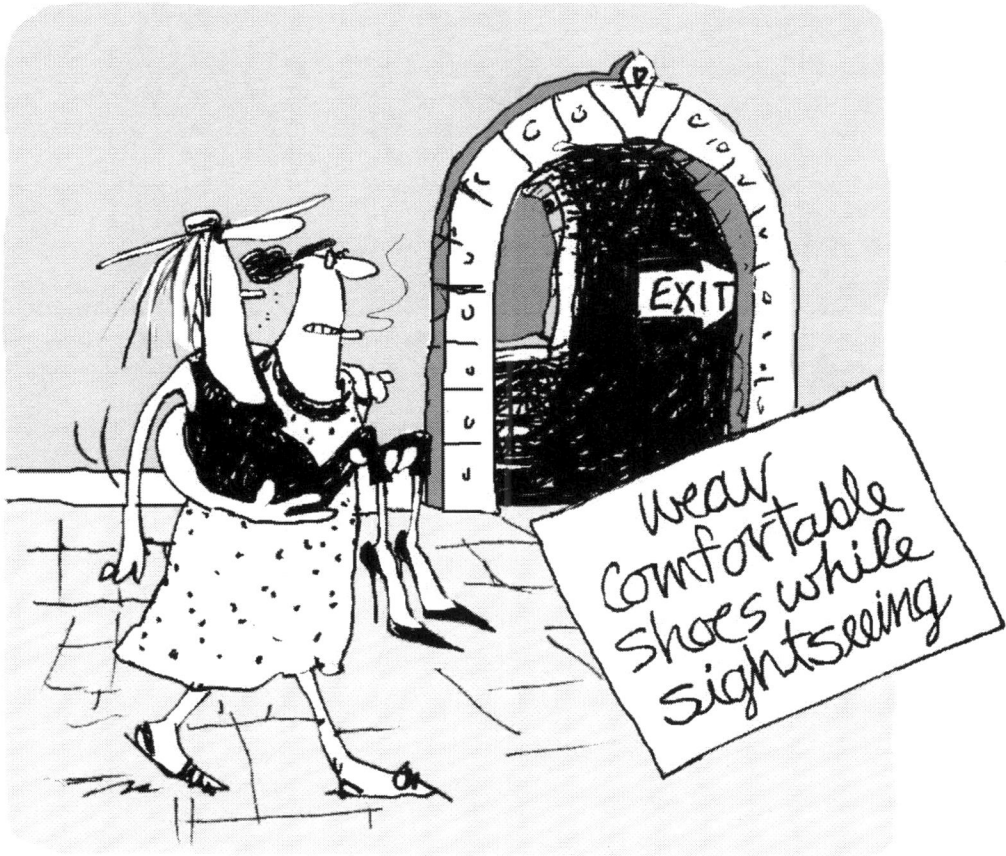

The most interesting places you can visit while traveling are usually just off the beaten track and make your trip so much more rewarding than slavishly following a guide map.

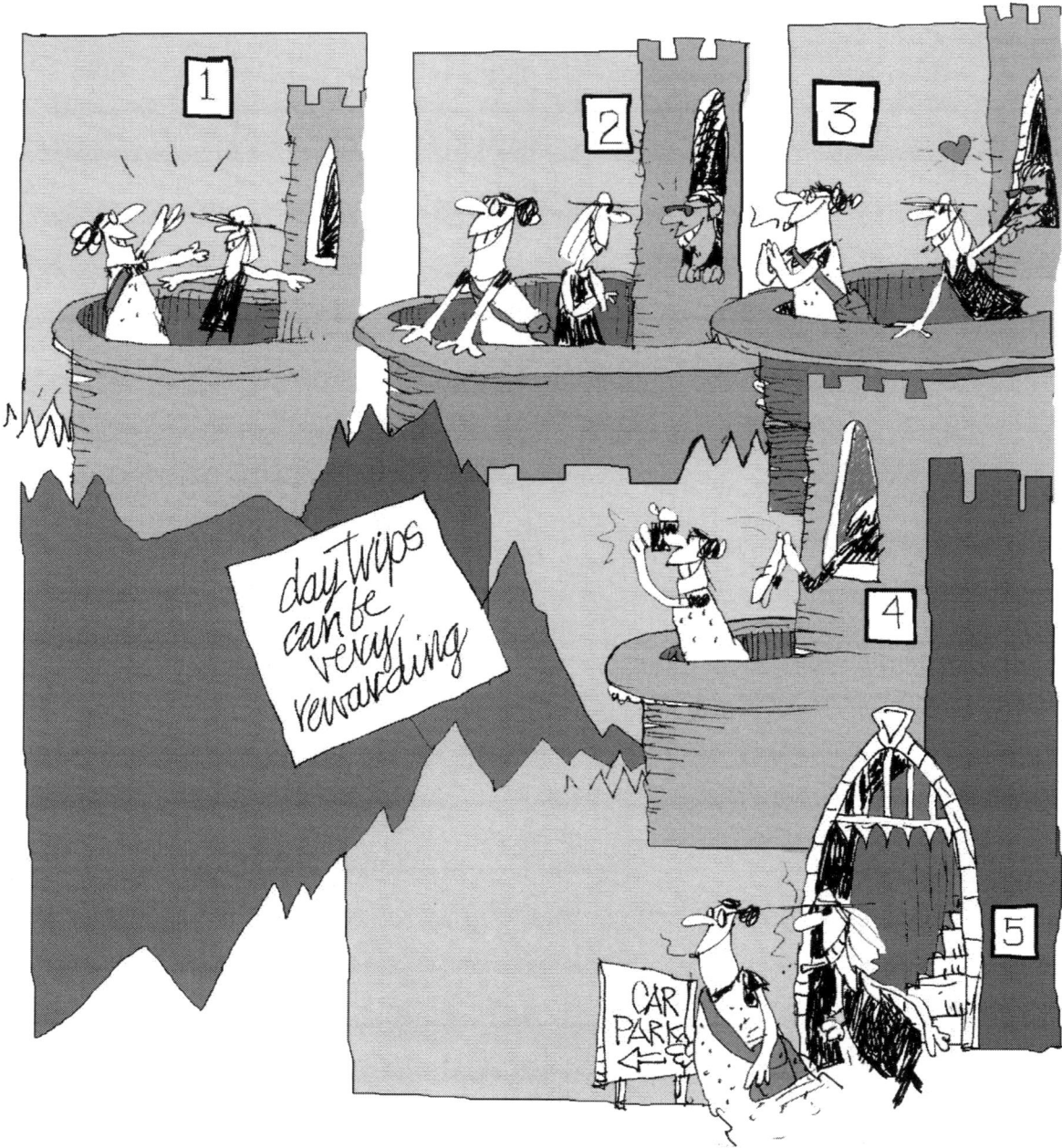

By only visiting a few sites (or even one) a day, you'll have time to really experience what you're seeing. Carefully looking at frescoed ceilings, columns or paintings is hard work; sometimes I feel like my eyes are just too full. If you cram too much into one outing you can easily become overloaded. Be honest with yourself and your companion. If you're overwhelmed or your pain is becoming unbearable, call it a day.

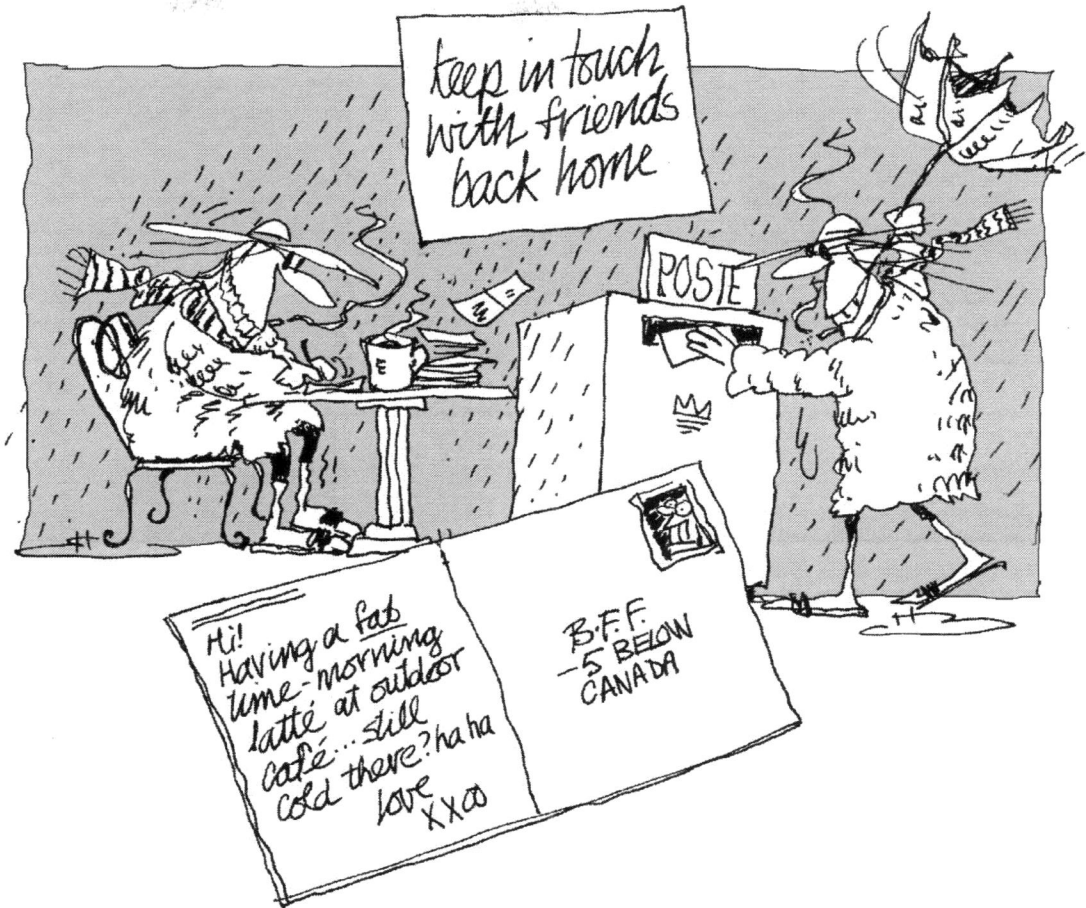

There's always tomorrow. Most often, you can go back if you need to see more, and if that's not possible, you've still seen more than you would have if you'd never left home.

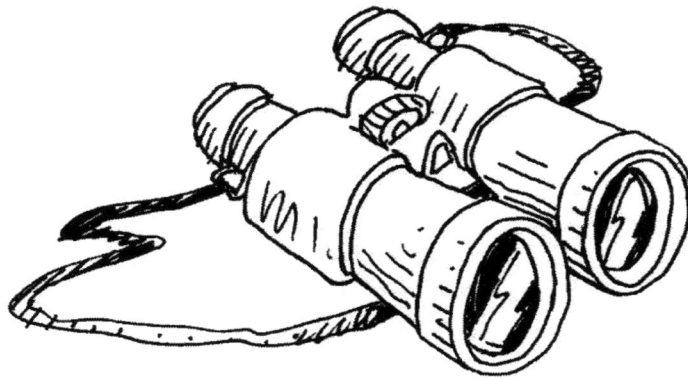

Chapter 8
SHOPPING

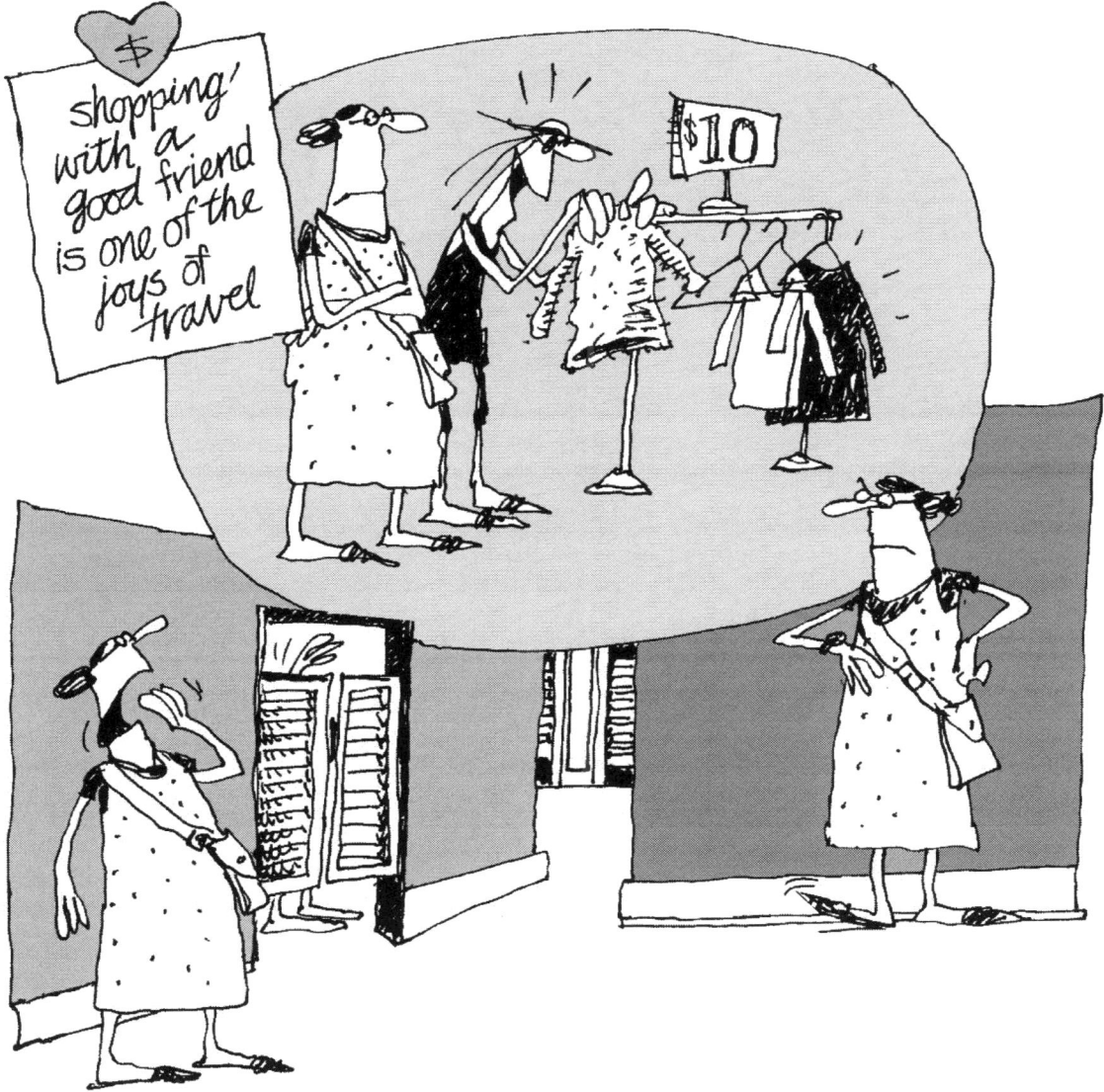

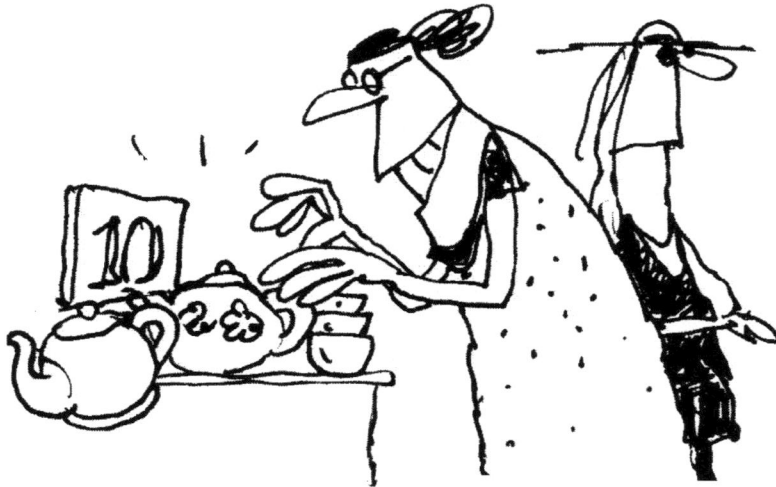

Shopping doesn't have to be an endurance test

Shopping is one of those things you either love or hate. If you really, really hate shopping, skip this chapter.

Now, let's deal with people who actually love poking around in markets and shops, finding little treasures for themselves and their long list of people at home.

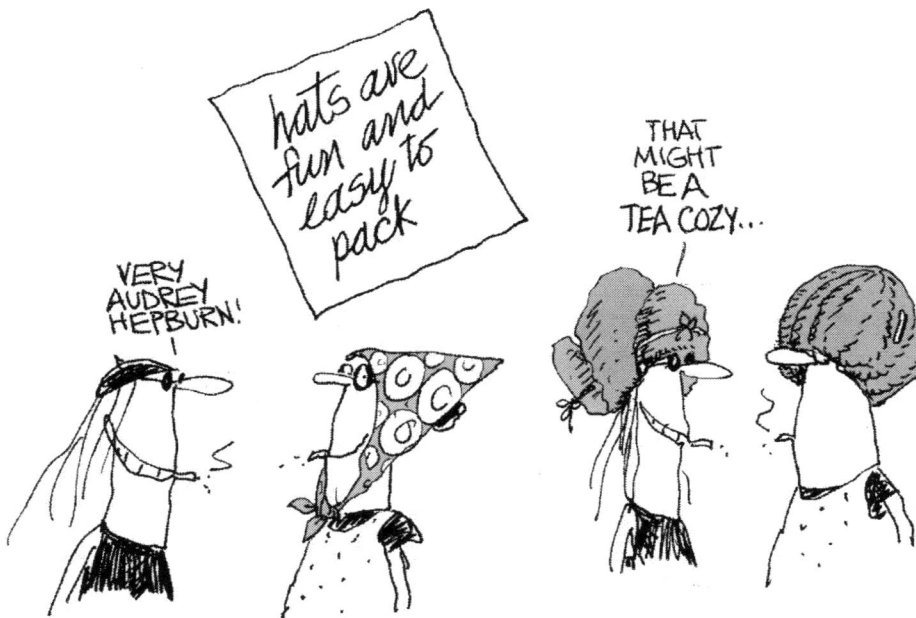

Plan, Plan, Plan!

Before you set out on a shopping trip, prepare for the attack and gather a few things together. A bit of pre-emptive planning can extend your outing and save significant frustration and pain.

Wear sensible shoes

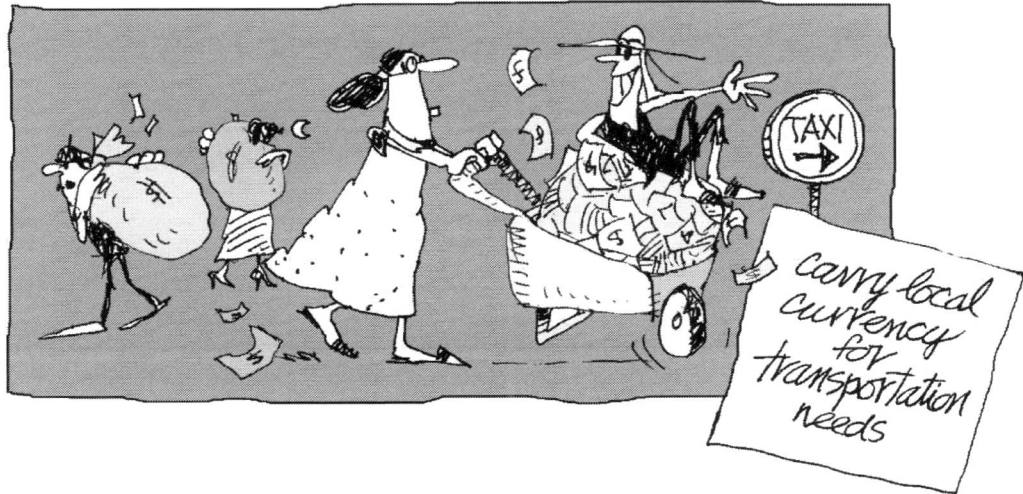

Bring a shopping bag with you—one of those nylon jobs that weighs nothing and folds into itself in your purse or pocket is perfect. They're capacious, lightweight and when full, act as a sign that it's probably time to stop shopping.

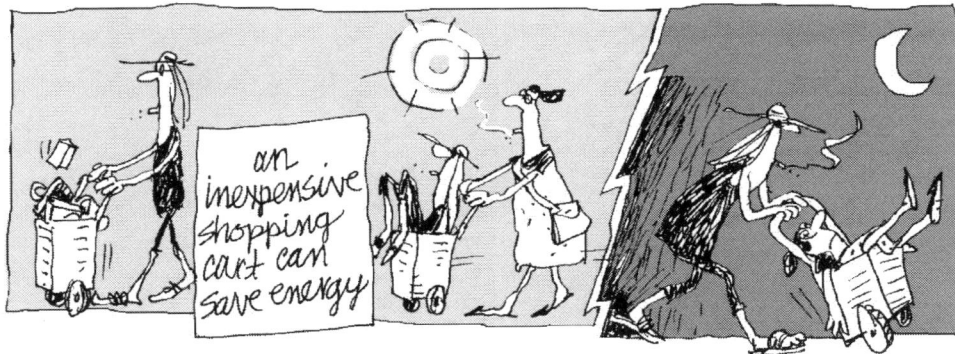

Don't leave "home" without the refillable water bottle you brought with you. Sometimes it's difficult to find potable water—and even if bottled water is readily available, you can feel good about being Green!

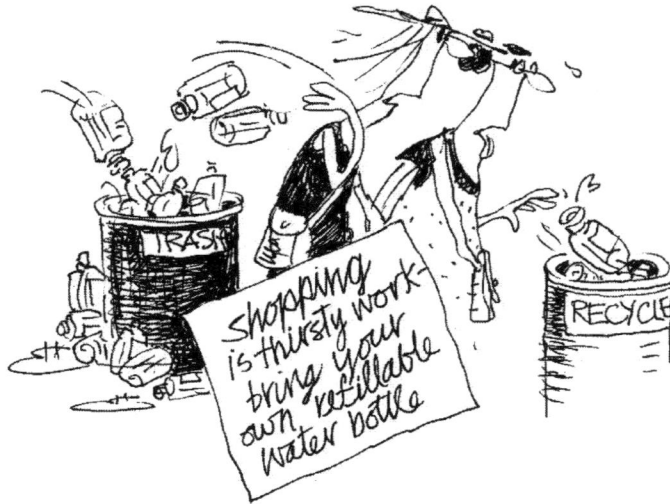

shopping is thirsty work- bring your own refillable water bottle

If it's too hot, plan to duck into air-conditioned stores or cafés whenever you can. If there's a mall you want to explore, take advantage of the climate-control and enjoy shopping in comfort on days when outdoor weather is inclement.

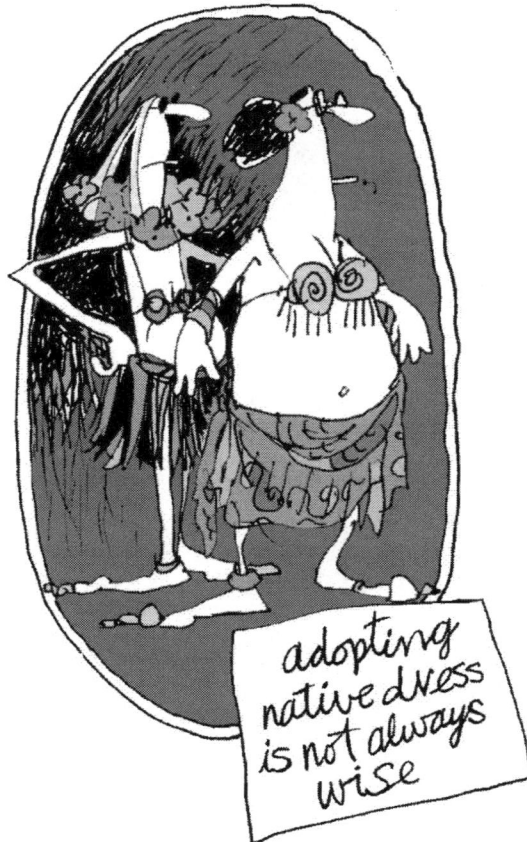

adopting native dress is not always wise

Set a time limit for shopping, especially if one of you has more endurance or interest than the other. Four hours (including travel time) is a reasonable limit and by pre-arranging this with your travel partner, you won't need to whine, plead, or feel guilty when it's time to quit.

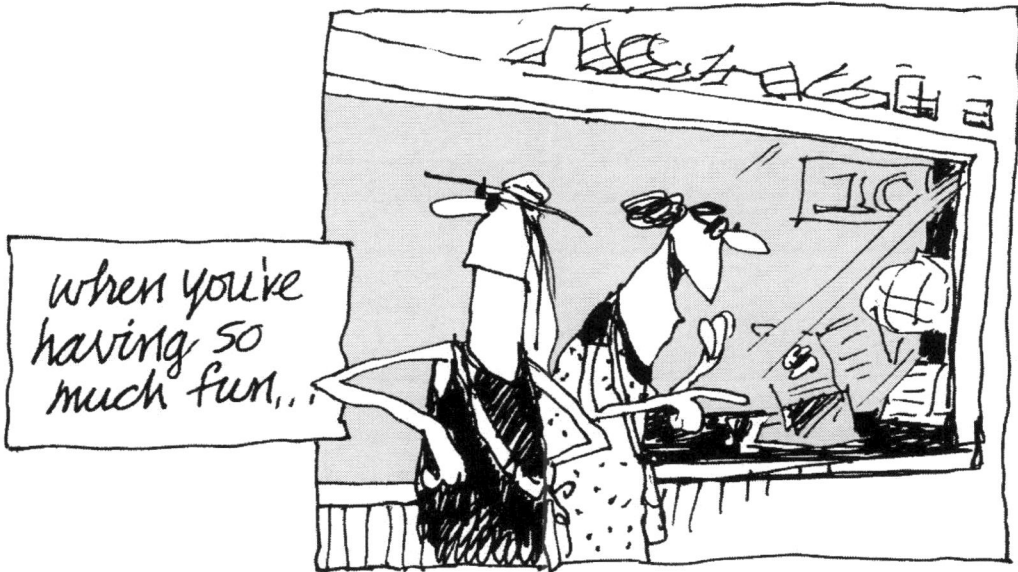

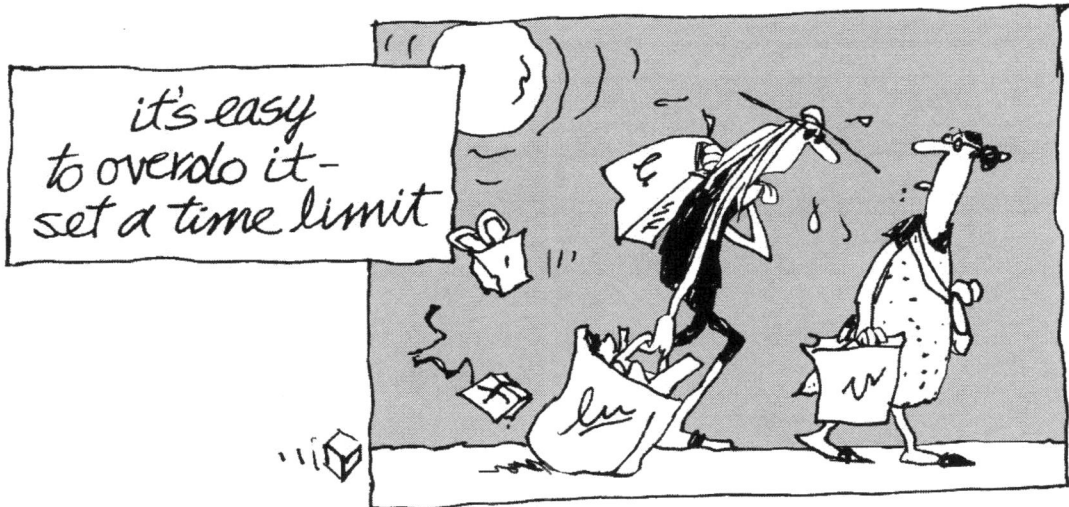

when you're having so much fun...

it's easy to overdo it— set a time limit

You Absolutely Must Have This!

Must you?

Don't stress yourself out over getting an absolutely different gift for everybody back home. If you find something lightweight and wonderful, get a bunch of them. If you can't find the perfect thing for someone, don't buy anything at all.

(If you're desperate for gifts, you could always have a look at the airport shops when leaving—maybe there's something there that would do. Or cheat. Go online and order something once you get home. Who will know if you don't say anything?)

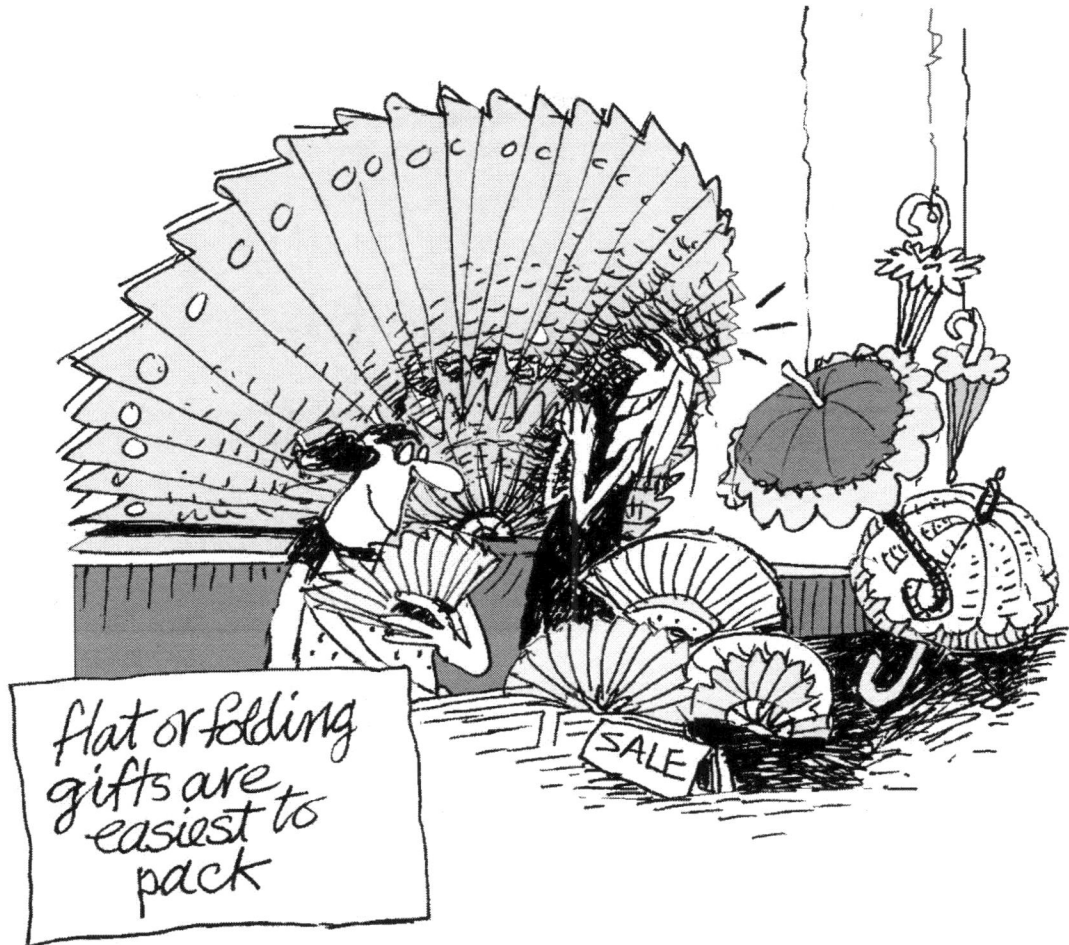

flat or folding
gifts are
easiest to
pack

Try not to buy heavy things. Pick purchases with an eye to size and weight. Will it fit in your suitcase? Will you have to buy another suitcase (and likely pay extra baggage fees) just to get it home? And if you must buy something ridiculously heavy and bulky, ask if the store can ship it home for you. If they can't or won't, you can take it to a shipping company and have it sent. Remember, though, if budget matters, you'll have to add the cost of shipping to your purchase.

If possible, buy the lightest items first. If you know you're going to buy a weighty book, come back to that store last, just before you catch a cab to your hotel or apartment. You don't want to carry excessively heavy bags around for hours. Even if you didn't have chronic pain, you'd have a backache by the end of the day.

If you're shopping in another country, it's a good idea to keep all your receipts in an envelope. When it comes time to fill out the customs form, you might not feel up to heavy arithmetic (or guesswork) at the border.

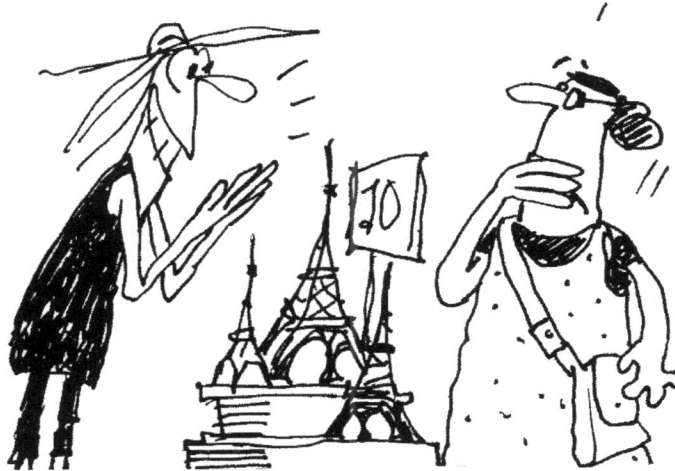

Most important shopping tip? Same as all the other advice in this book: pace yourself. Pause for a while every half hour or so. Sit on a bench and watch the people go by, sit at an outdoor café while enjoying a coffee or snack, sit on the grass and chat—whatever you do, a short break will help you continue your outing with renewed energy.

So have a great time, don't wear yourself out and don't stress. Remember: vacation shopping is supposed to be fun.

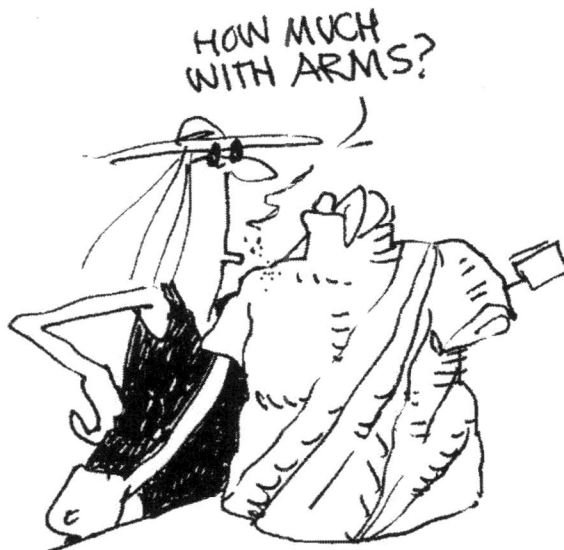

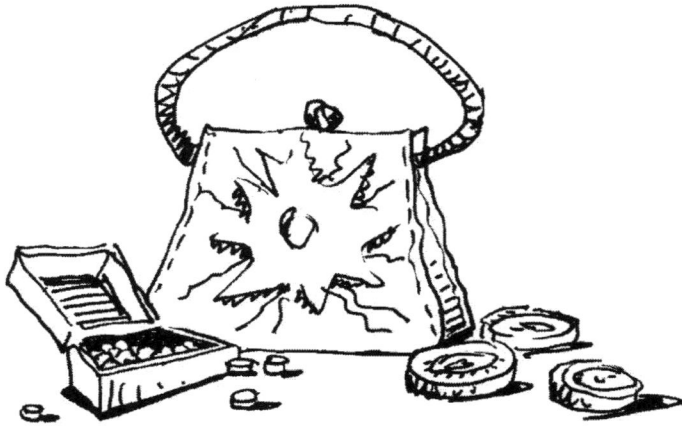

Chapter 9
ADAPTABILITY

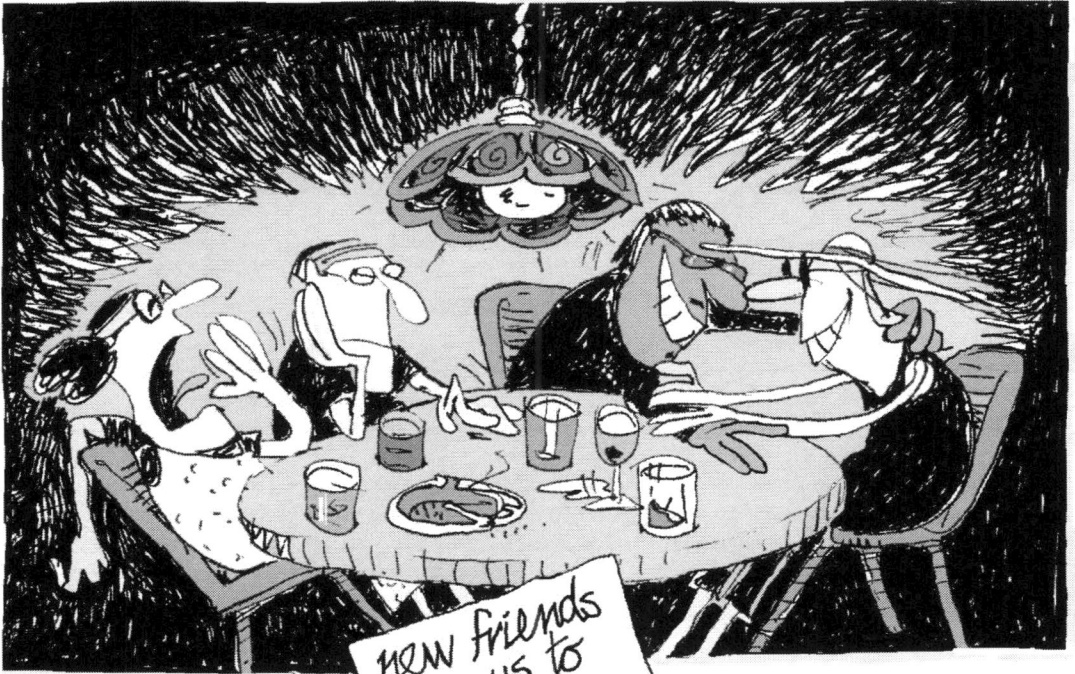

new friends open us to new experiences

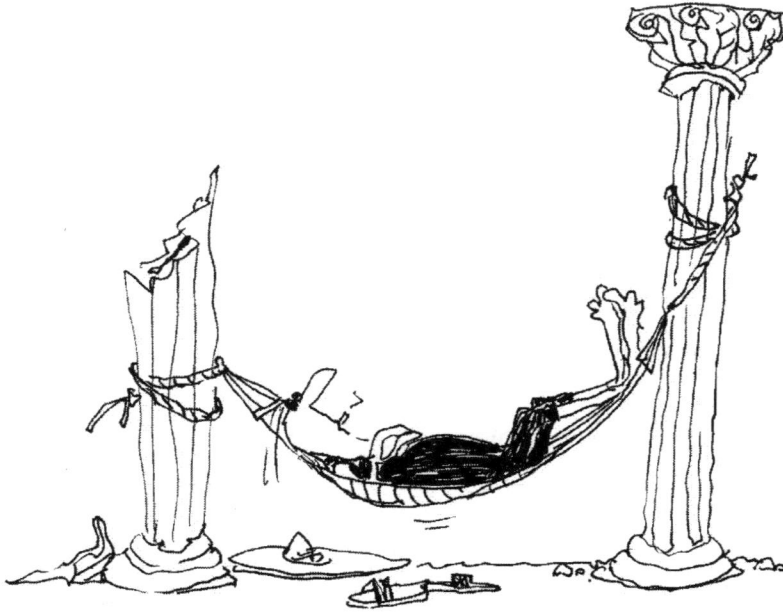

A little research will often allay your travel fears

One of the hardest things to do when traveling is to adapt to different time zones and cultures. It's difficult, if not impossible, to completely fit into another culture, but some adaptation will make your stay much pleasanter and make you a more welcome visitor.

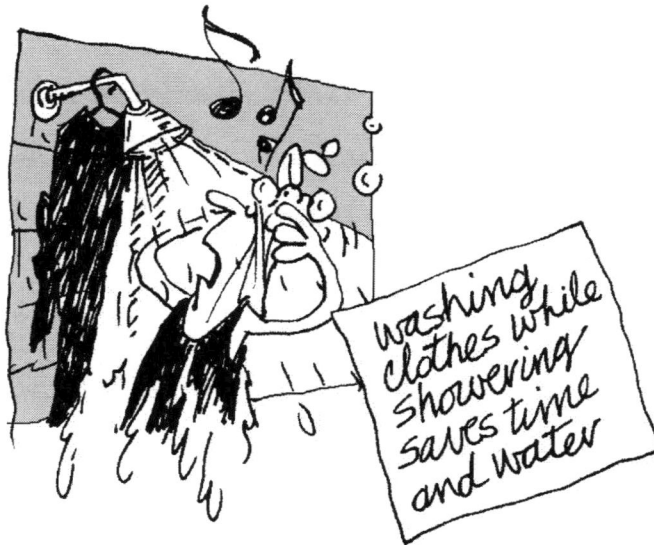

washing clothes while showering saves time and water

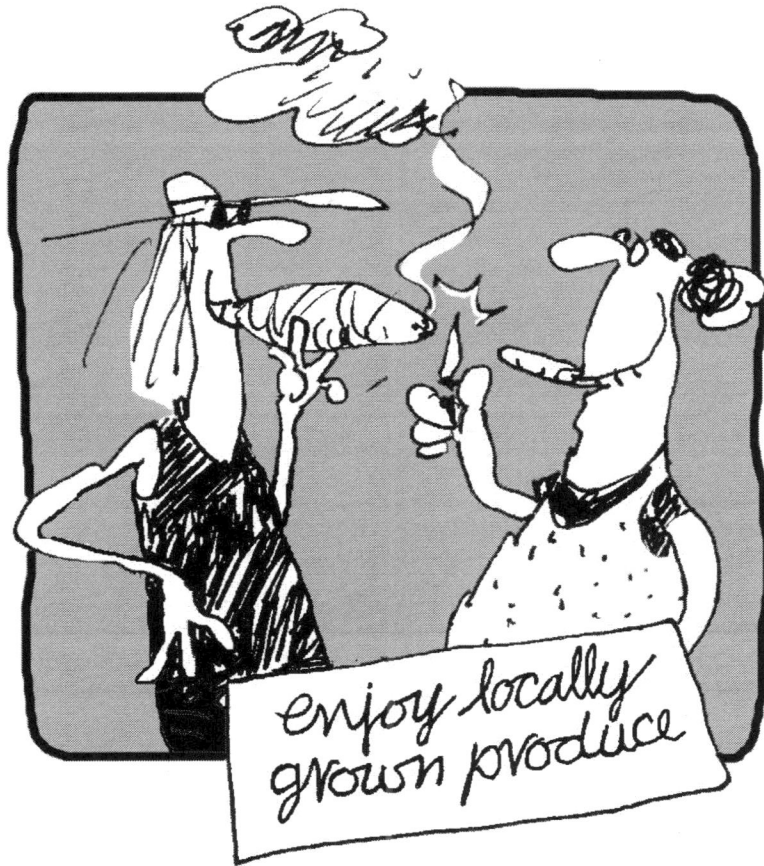

enjoy locally grown produce

In terms of fitting in, a traveler with chronic pain isn't that different from the regular tourist. Unfortunately, the need for help arises more often for us, and in that unwelcome situation, some knowledge of local customs will come in handy.

What if you need to seek medical help when the entire country takes a nap or eats its main meal between two and four in the afternoon? Knowing that it's easier to find a doctor in the morning and later in the afternoon or early evening can help you to plan. Knowing how to contact emergency help can save your life.

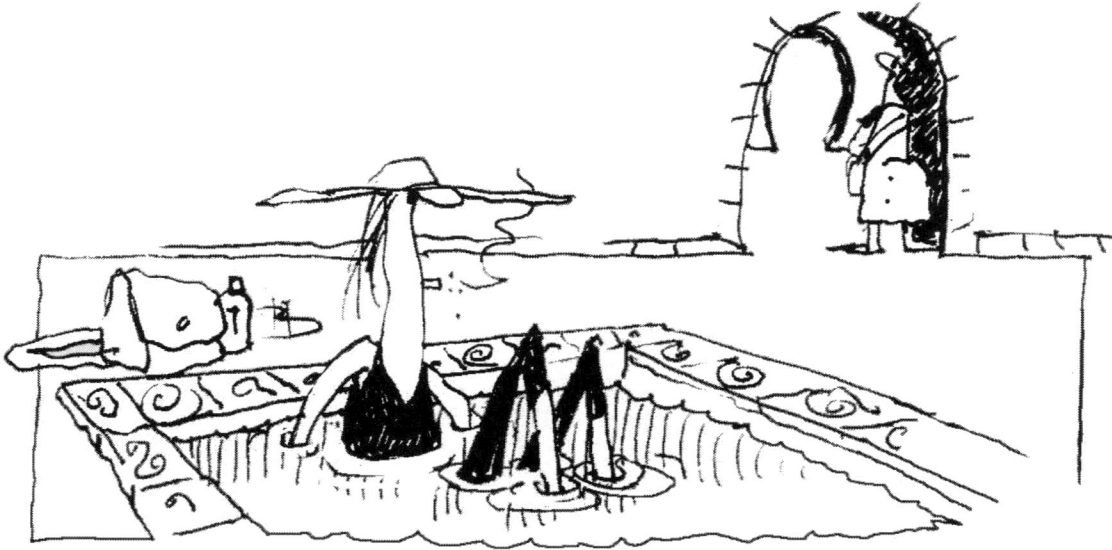

When extremes of temperature affect your pain levels, make some allowance for that when you're wandering about:

Carry a folding fan

Bring drinking water

Wear a hat in very hot places

Dress appropriately in layers

Wear warm clothing for very cold places.

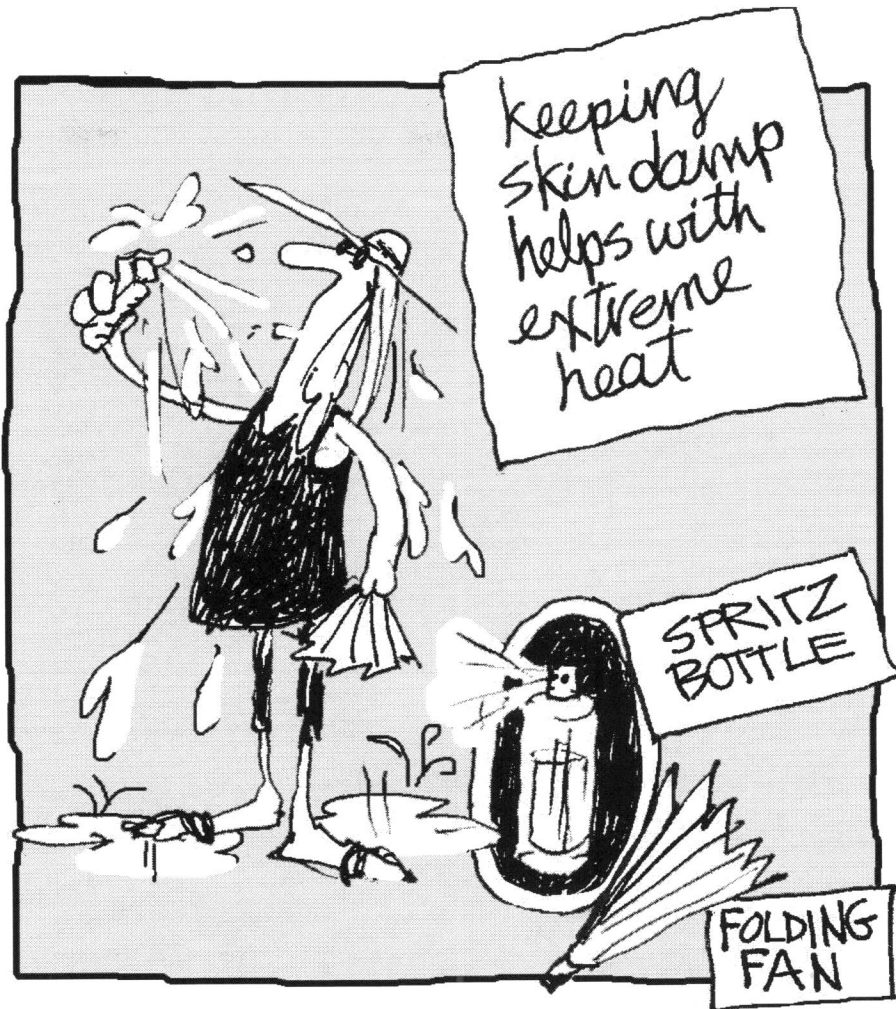

Find out how the locals deal with the extremes. Although they're used to it and you're not, they might have some tips or suggestions to help you cope. Most importantly, abide by the local customs on when to go out and when to stay in. Even people born to extreme temperatures pay attention to optimum times for work, rest and play. Their culture will reflect it.

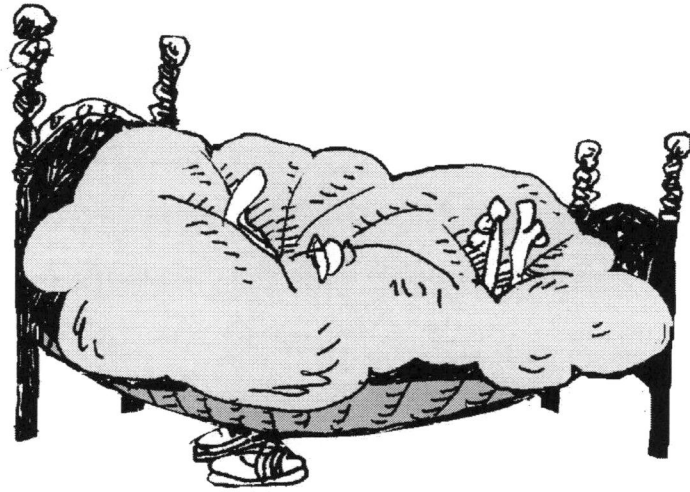

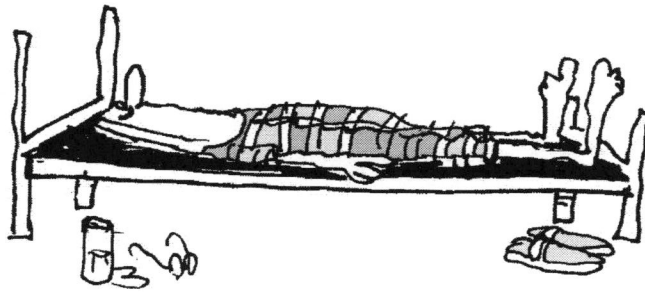

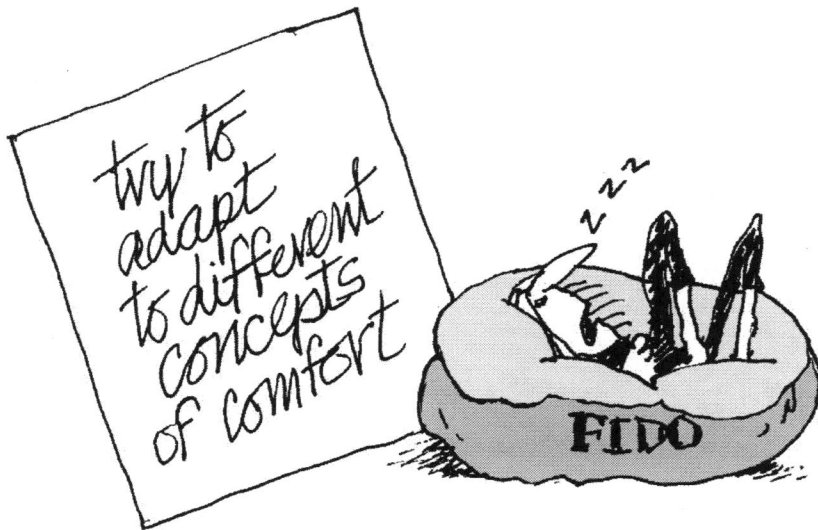

If it's important that you eat regular meals, find out when restaurants and cafés open and close; for example, most restaurants in Europe close after lunch and stay closed, often till seven, but in Mexico, since many families still share their main meal from 2 to 4 pm, virtually all restaurants are open. If you're starving at 5:30 because you haven't adapted to your host country's meal times and haven't bought any groceries, you'll have a long, uncomfortable wait till you eat again.

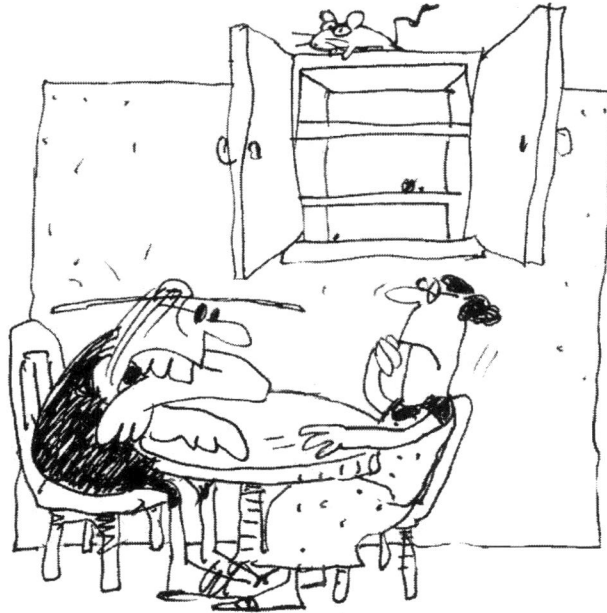

While many people in other countries speak English, especially in major cities, this is not always so in the countryside. A smattering of phrases in the other language will go a long way toward making you more welcome (not to mention getting you the service you require). Phrase books are handy; electronic translators even more so. It's polite to at least know "please" and "thank you" in your host country's language.

Shopping is often different than you're used to. In hot-weather countries, stores close in the heat of the afternoon but open again when it's cooler and stay open late. In those places, the evening is the preferred time to shop, eat and promenade, and it's great fun to join in.

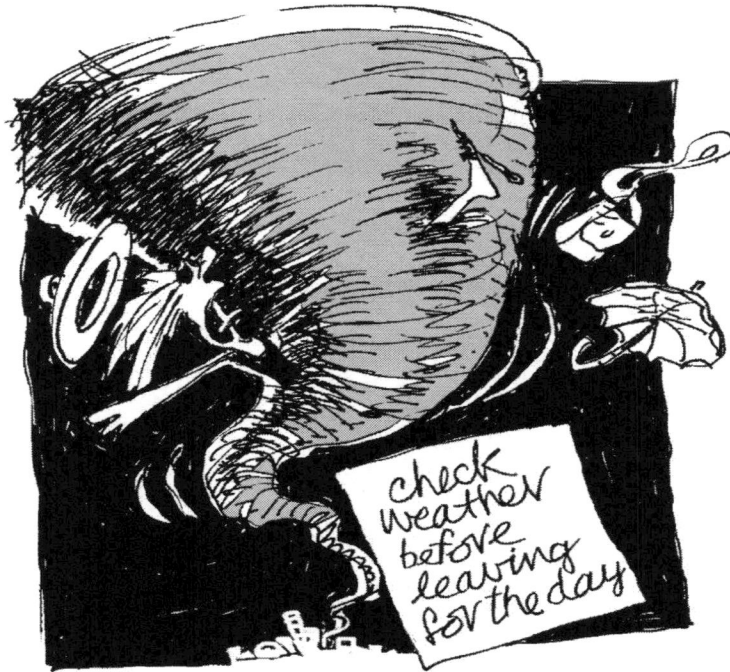

If your stomach has been trained for years in the Western tradition of three squares a day, it's handy if you have a fridge where you can stock a few snacks while you're adapting. A kettle or coffee pot in the room is always welcome. You can make coffee or tea when the rest of the world is napping. After a few days, you'll be used to the different culture and enjoy an afternoon siesta before lingering over a meal in your favorite café long into the evening.

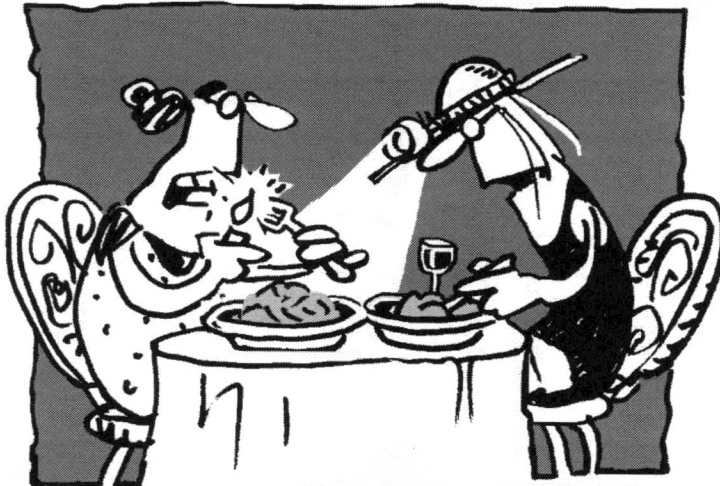

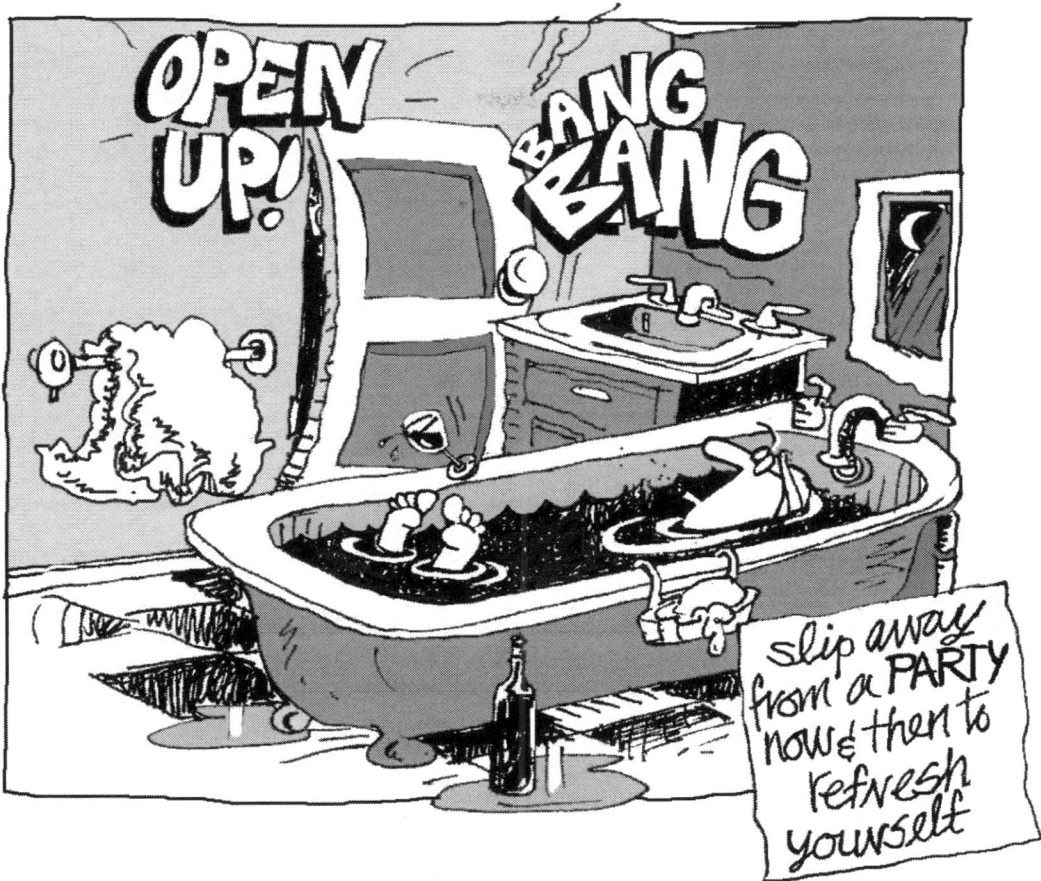

In Cuba, where my friend Sheryl lived for a year, parties start late and go on for a long time (her birthday party lasted 24 hours!!!). It's totally acceptable to drop out of the party, find a place in the host's home to rest, and then rejoin the party later.

Although Western dress is tolerated almost everywhere, in some countries it's more considerate to at least make a nod to their customs. Covering your hair (for women) in churches or not wearing shorts on the street is easy and shows respect to your hosts. Again, a little research ahead of time will stand you in good stead on arrival. And it's always fun to shop for a bit of local clothing to jazz up your wardrobe.

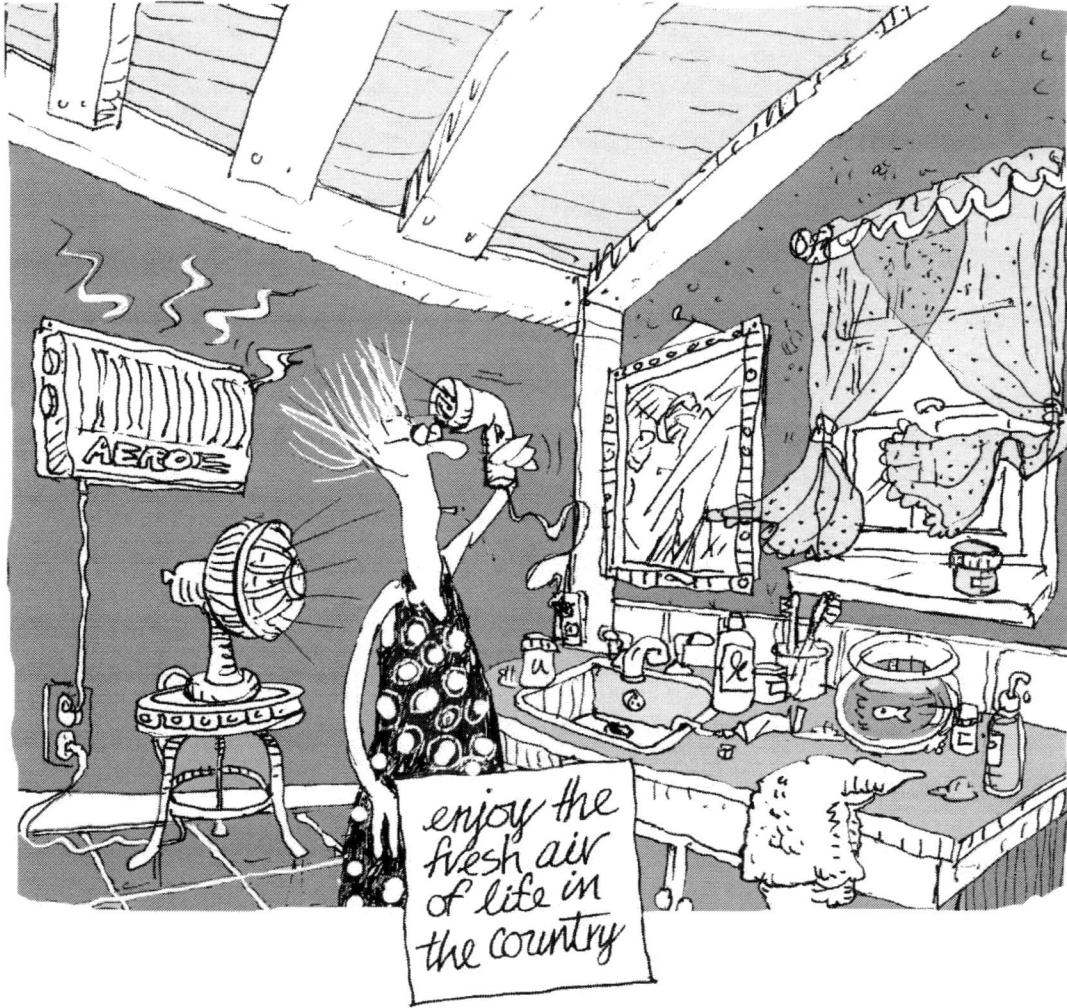

enjoy the
fresh air
of life in
the country

Altogether, it's more fun to adapt to a new culture as much as possible. Why visit another country if we just drag our own iron-clad habits around with us?

Soon you'll be taking a siesta every afternoon, sipping sundowners at twilight and eating fashionably late every evening. What better souvenir to bring home from your travels than a welcome change of routine?

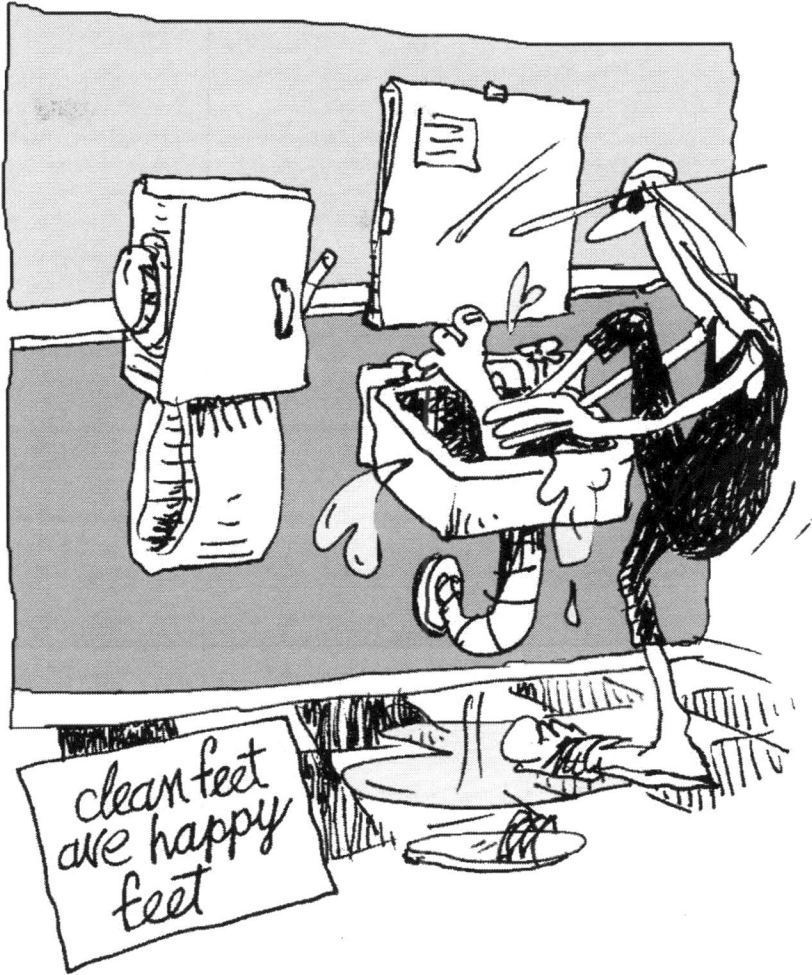

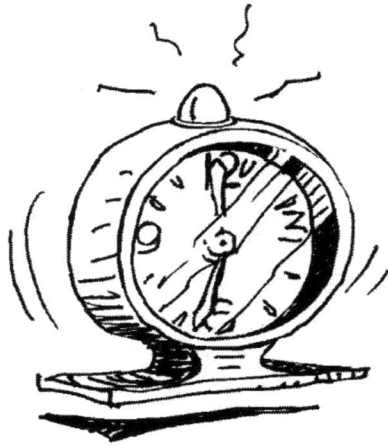

Chapter 10
BATHROOM CUSTOMS

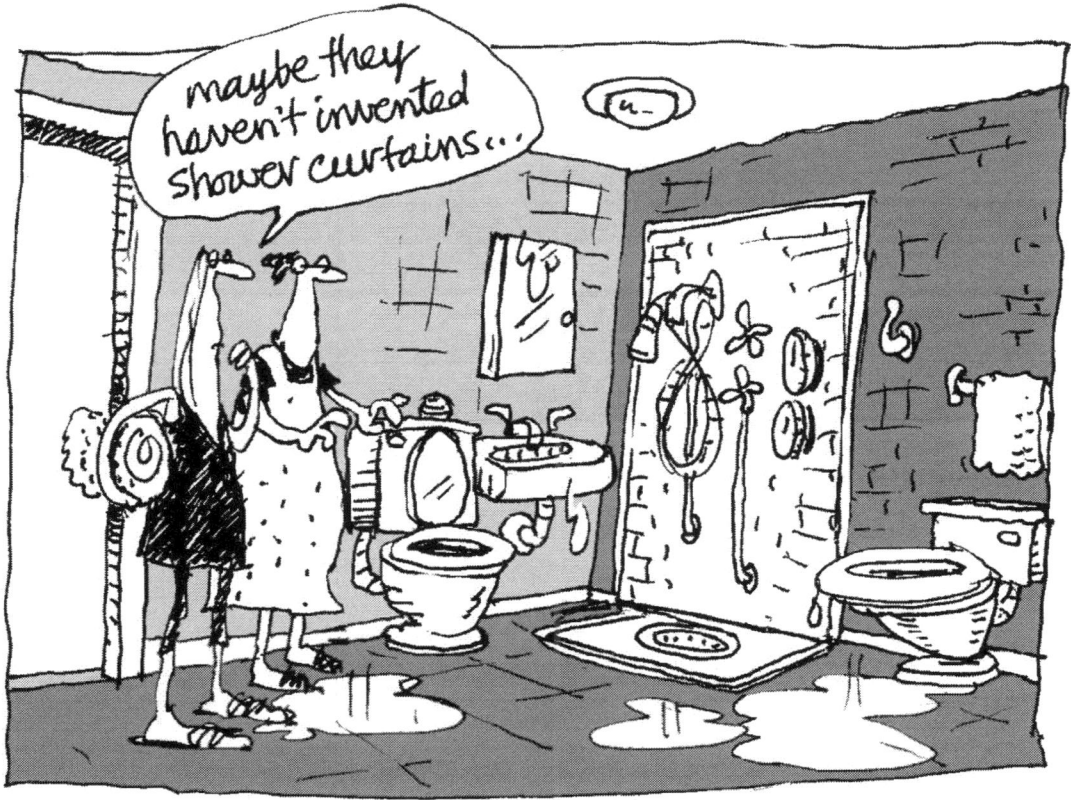

maybe they haven't invented shower curtains...

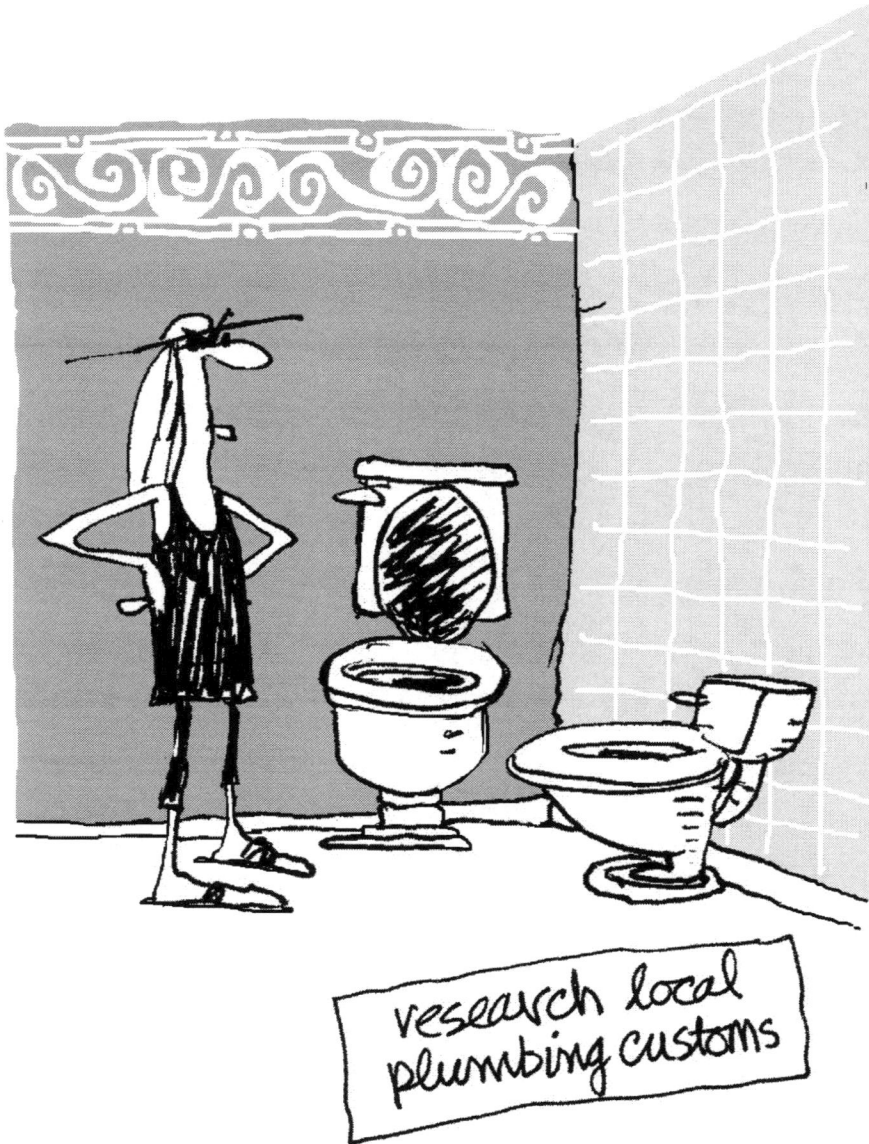

Know how to find — and use — the bathroom

Given our basic human needs, you'd think toilets would be much the same throughout the world, but since technology developed more quickly in some places and seemingly not at all in others, the toilet is not standard issue.

From a hole in the floor to a high-tech, wash 'n' dry wonder, a travel book dedicated solely to The Toilet would not be amiss.

Just as toilets vary, so too do customs surrounding the use of the toilet.

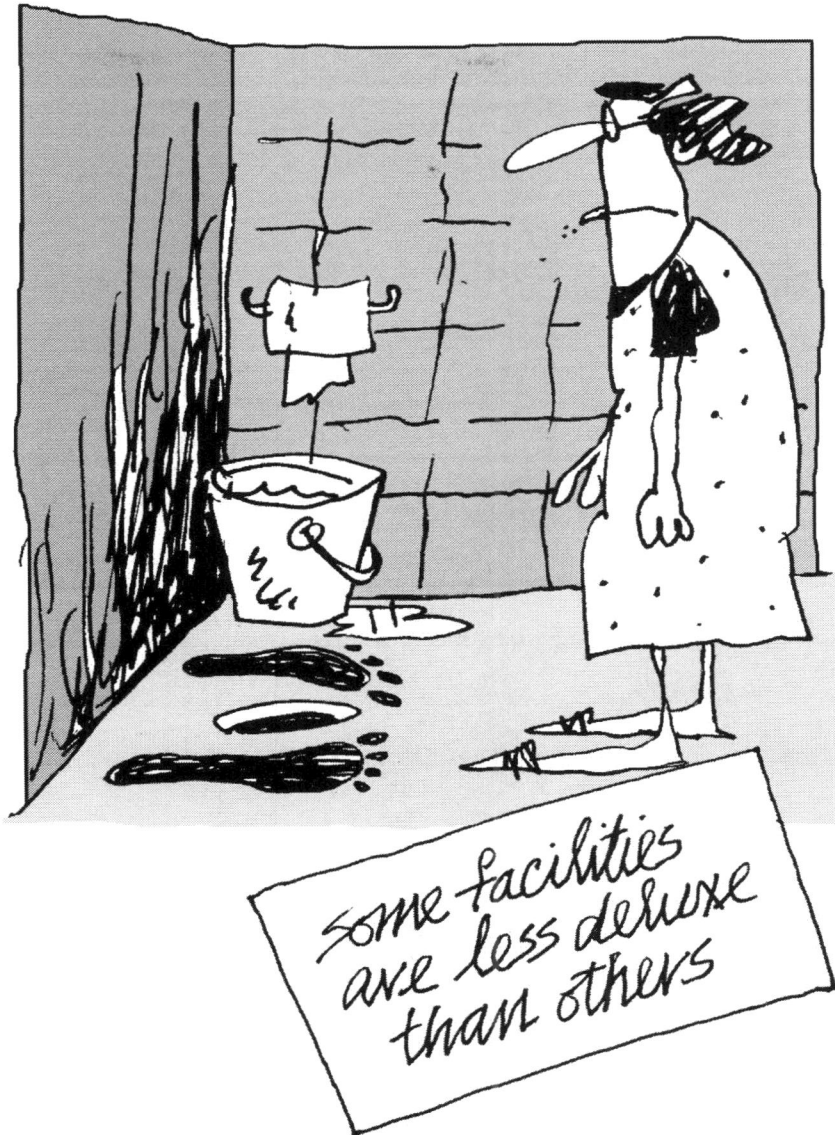

some facilities are less deluxe than others

One of the problems with chronic pain is that painkillers are often also diuretics, so locating—and understanding—the nearest toilet is a serious concern. A little research before you leave can save you time and embarrassment and make your stay in a foreign locale much easier.

If you're often in need of a toilet, learn the phrase "Where is the washroom?" in the dominant language of the country you're visiting. In every language course, almost the first thing they teach you is, "Where is the bathroom?" — clearly, it's a useful phrase. People will usually know from your accent that you're not a native and simply point, rather than go on and on with a verbal answer you couldn't possibly interpret. Don't be embarrassed. You're not the first visitor, or the last, with an urgent bladder but at least you were able to ask. Sometimes mime is not appropriate.

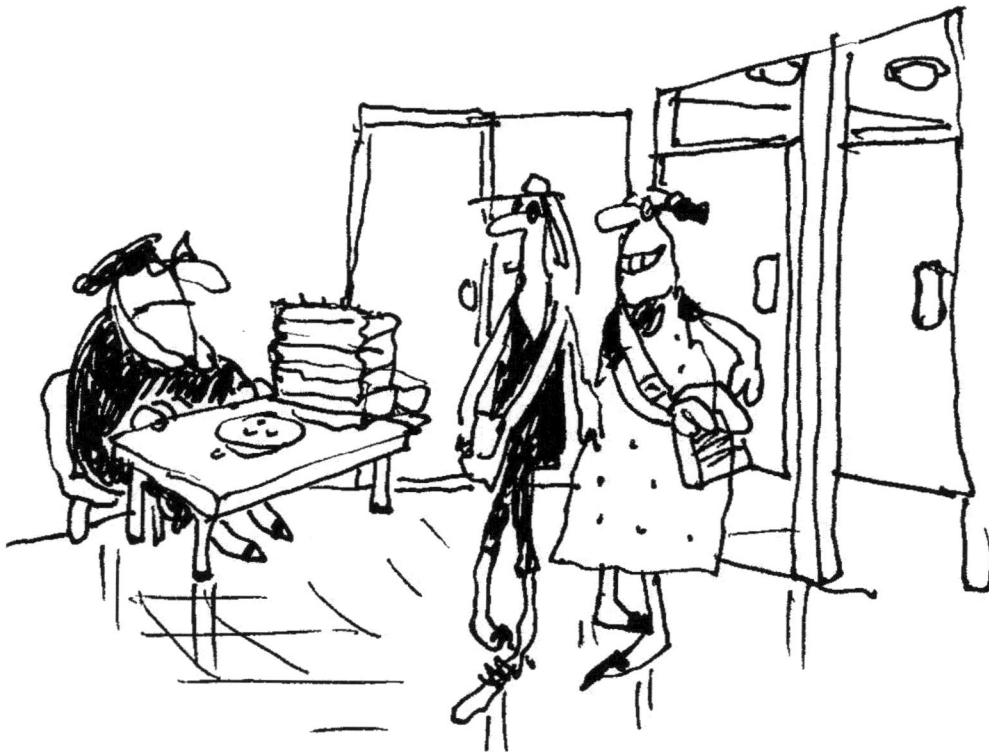

In many places, you'll find an attendant in the washroom. You don't have to pay this person who hands you squares of toilet paper, a towel at the wash basin or bobby pins to tuck up your hair, but it's embarrassing if you don't have any coins for her in your pocket.

Just as with toilets, bathing systems also vary widely. Some showers in the UK need an engineering degree to manipulate. You might even come across, as I once did in a B & B in Bath of all places, a weird contraption similar in its way to the Murphy Bed. This proudly advertised, fold-up shower-in-the-room was beyond my ability even to open, much less operate.

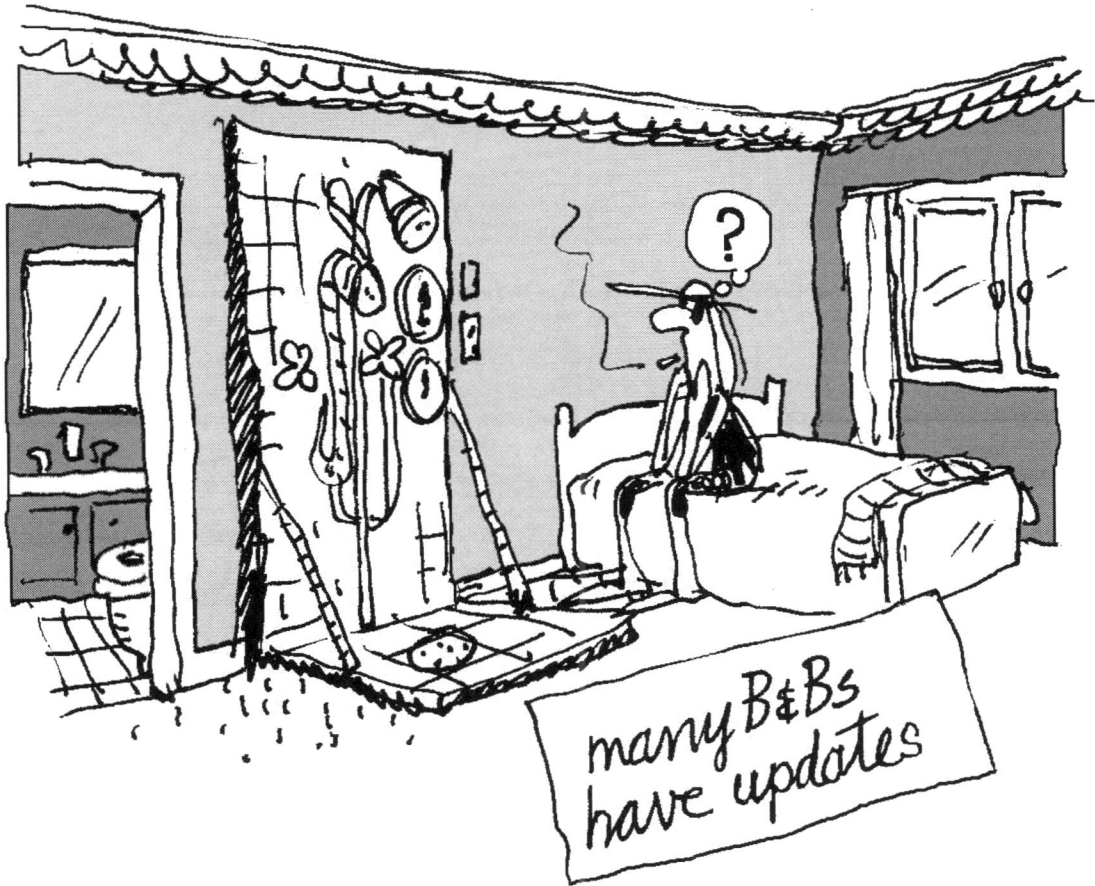

many B&Bs
have updates

But perhaps this isn't accidental. Hot water costs money. The more tourists who don't actually avail themselves of the shower, the more money in the innkeeper's pocket. Again, a little research on your accommodation ahead of time could save you frustration later.

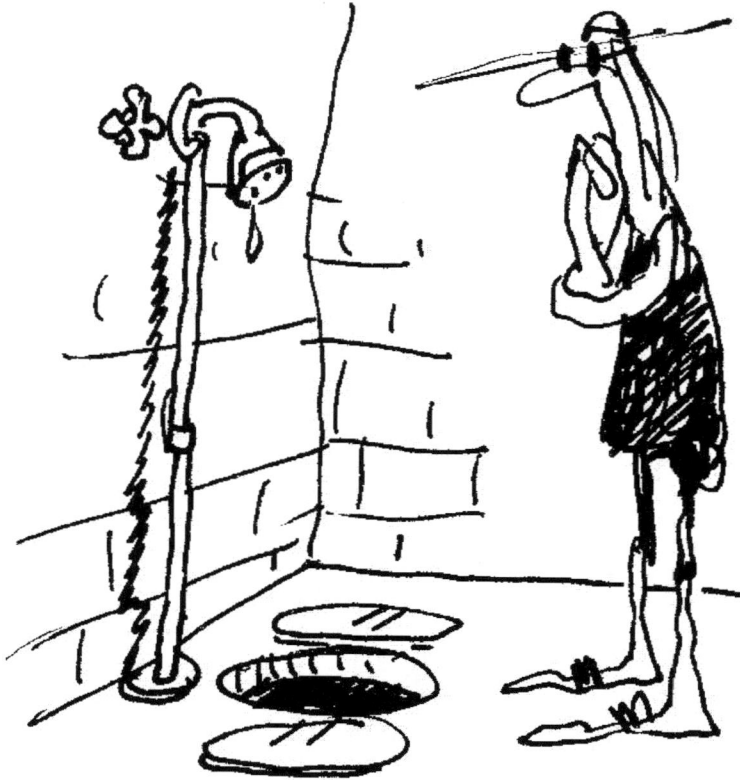

Toilets, showers and bathtubs in major cities are becoming more alike as the world becomes increasingly standardized, but any trip you take that's even a bit off the tourist grid will land you in bathrooms you'll be telling your friends about later.

Customs and habits vary as well. Our North American insistence on separate washrooms for men and women is not always the norm. Bidets, still a rarity in our hotels and apartments, are standard issue in many European countries.

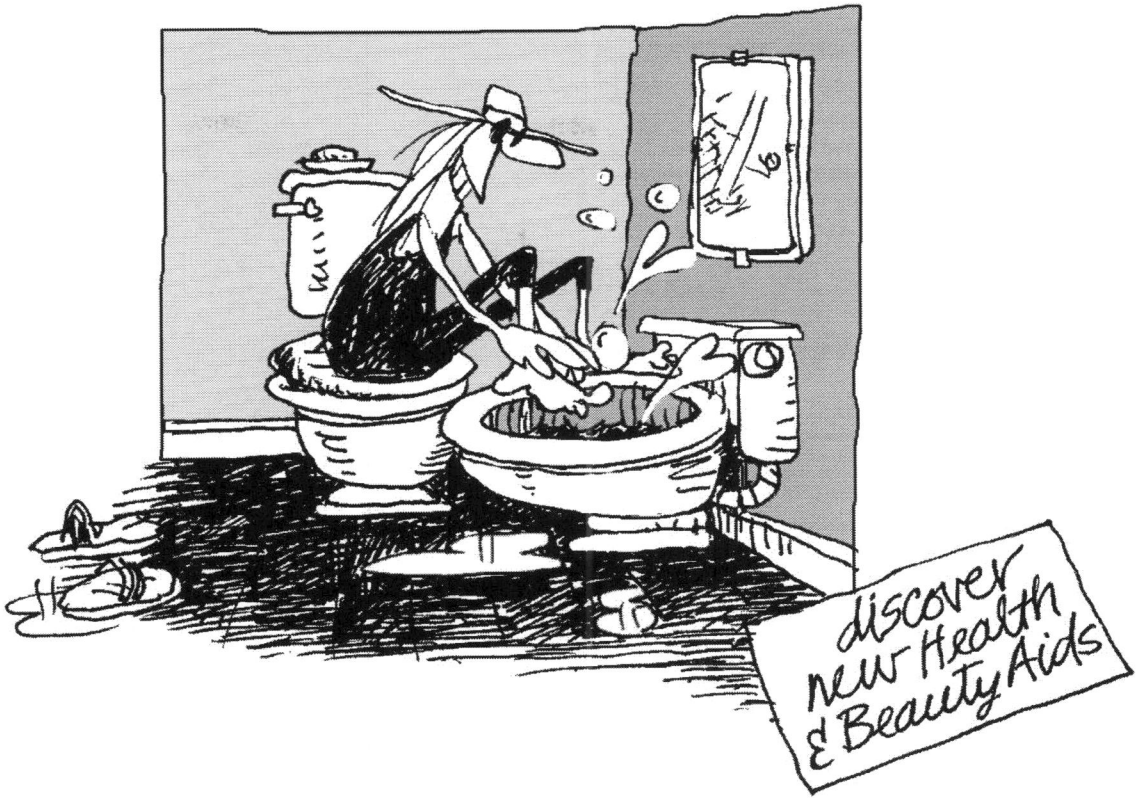

In some parts of the world where orthodox faiths are widely practiced, there is often an etiquette regarding personal hygiene when using the toilet that it may be advisable to know. The Internet can provide helpful, location-specific info on this subject.

If you're traveling to the Middle East, be advised that Muslims consider the left hand unclean. Don't use it for eating, shaking hands or offering gifts. Custom requires that the left hand is used in the toilet. No amount of hand washing afterwards will make it acceptable for social use.

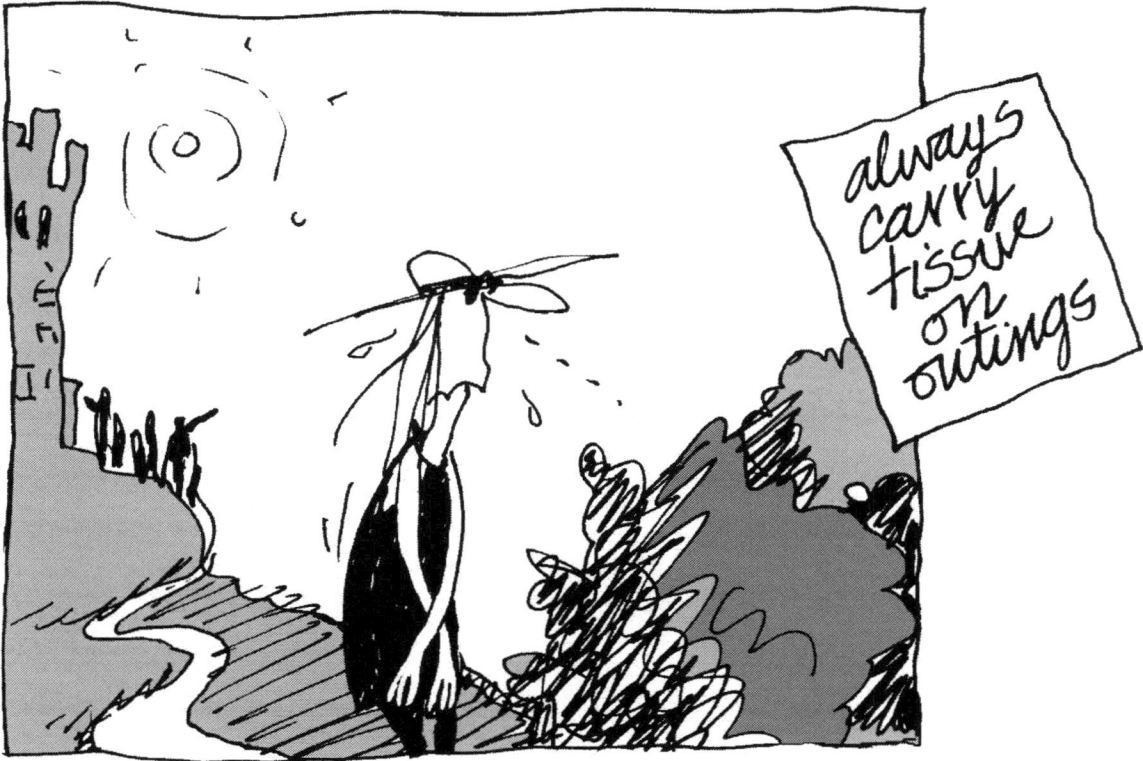

Toilet paper, though almost always available in tourist areas, is not necessarily provided when venturing off the beaten track. In some places, if your sensitive nether region requires the soft touch of three-ply, pack your own.

In the improbable event that you find yourself deep in the Arabian Desert after a hard day lurching along atop a camel and suddenly the spicy food you ate in the tent last night is demanding an immediate exit, don't be too surprised if instead of toilet paper you're offered a small pile of rounded rocks. Three is the usual number. Be cheered by the fact that when the Shamal blows, nasty bits of used tissue won't be whipping around—it's unlikely that anyone will be accidentally smacked in the face by a used rock.

If there's no certainty of a sink in the public washrooms, a small bottle of hand sanitizer in your bag will come in handy.

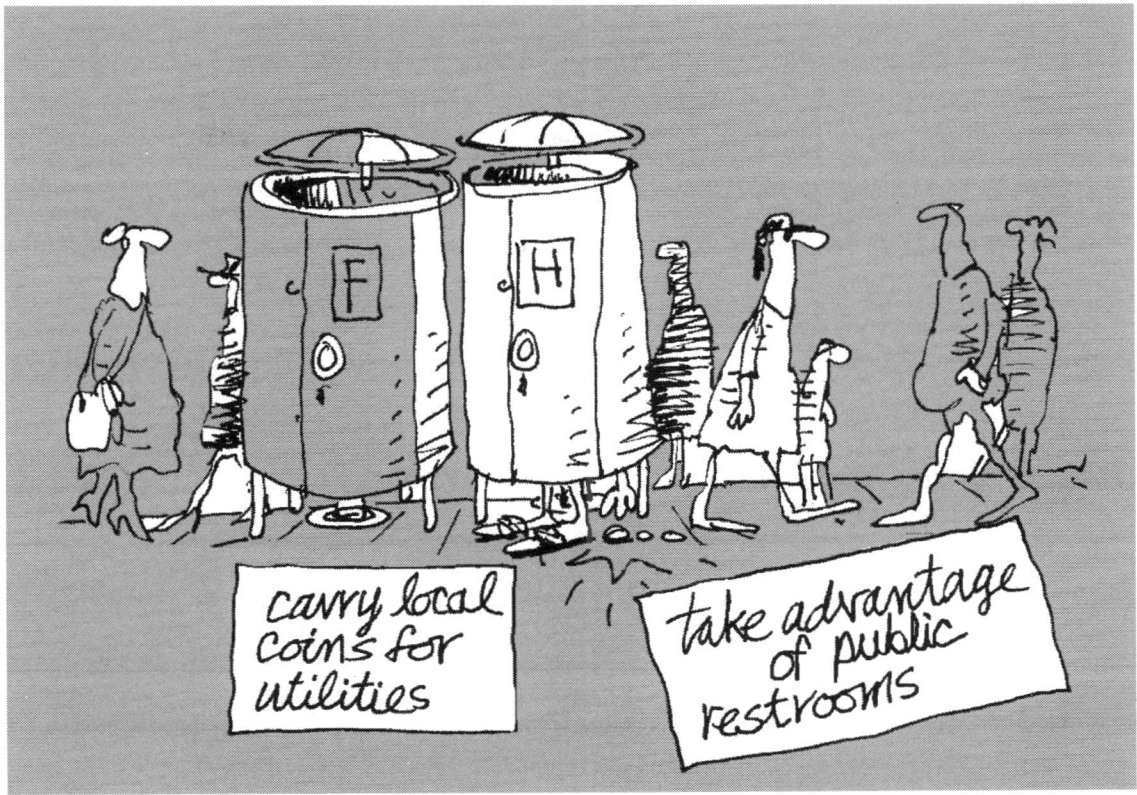

However strange it seems at first, rest assured: from the incredibly primitive to the sleekly futuristic, there always have been and always will be bathrooms. Your needs will be met.

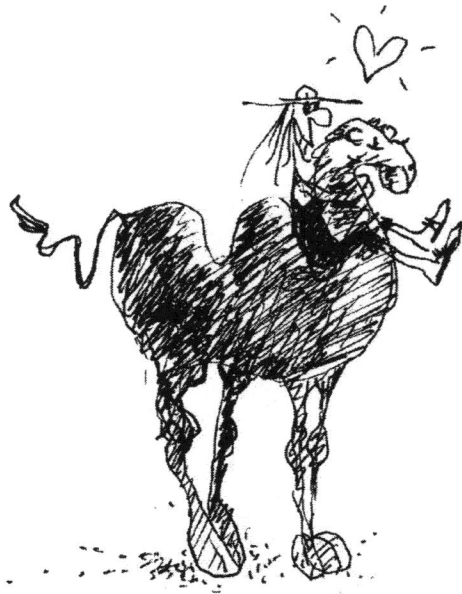

Chapter 11
NOBODY'S PERFECT

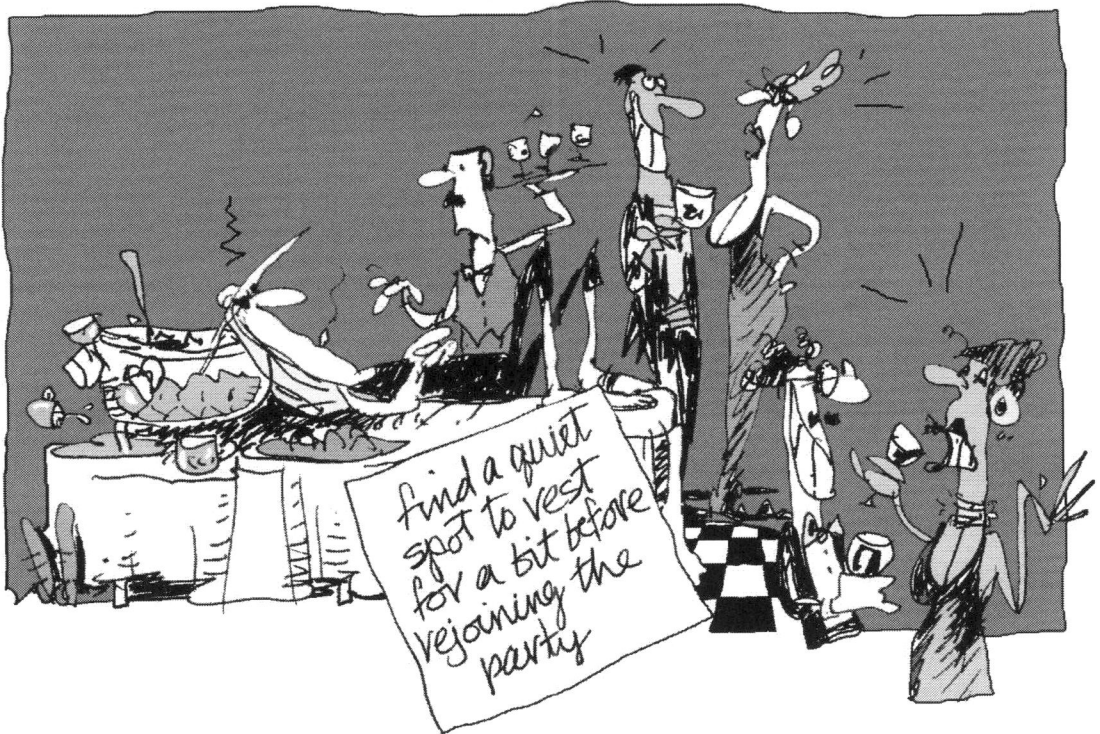

find a quiet spot to rest for a bit before rejoining the party

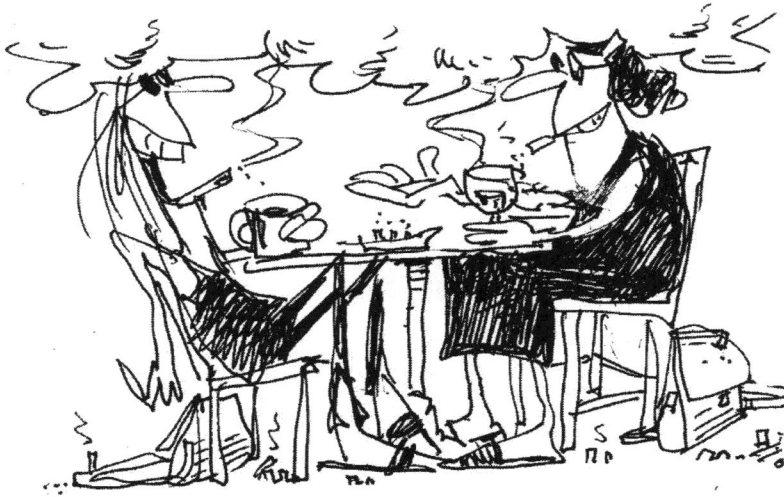

Suffering from chronic pain is no guarantee of good behavior

A strange thing occasionally comes over people living with chronic pain—often intensified by travel—and that's the feeling that you should somehow, magically, be able to live like other people. And sometimes you feel as though you should actually be rewarded for putting up with pain no one else has to suffer.

But nobody said life would be fair (and if they did, they're just wrong). You already know that rewarding yourself with ordinary self-indulgences (overeating, over-drinking, smoking, staying up too late . . . the list could fill a book) will almost always exacerbate the pain, but most of us, from time to time, do it anyway, especially when we're traveling. Even those without chronic pain often leave their best judgment at home.

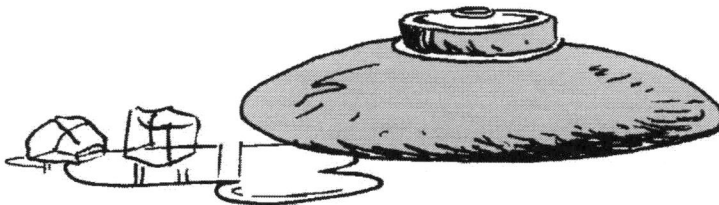

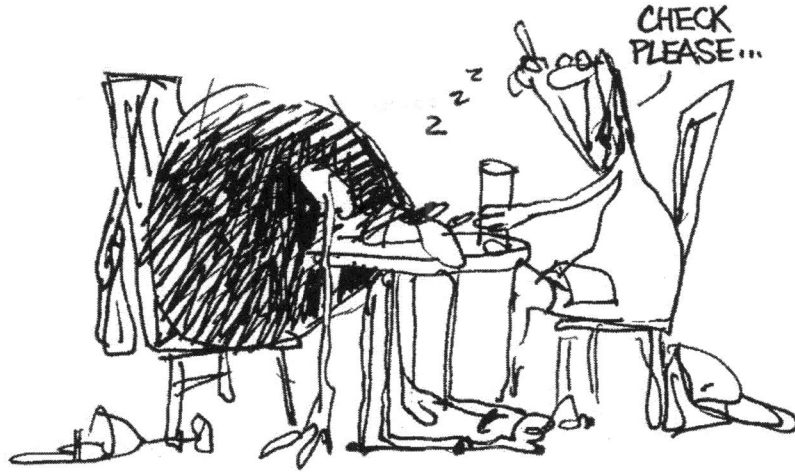

Everyone falls off a wagon or two when they're traveling. You just have to know how to land. Travelers eat and drink too much, ignore diets, walk too far, engage in unwise sexual behavior, stay up too late and mix up their medications. An error in judgment will almost certainly happen if you're having any fun at all. Just try really hard not to let the mistakes pile up for too long or you'll end up in a major meltdown. Have fun, but plan to fall back and regroup now and then.

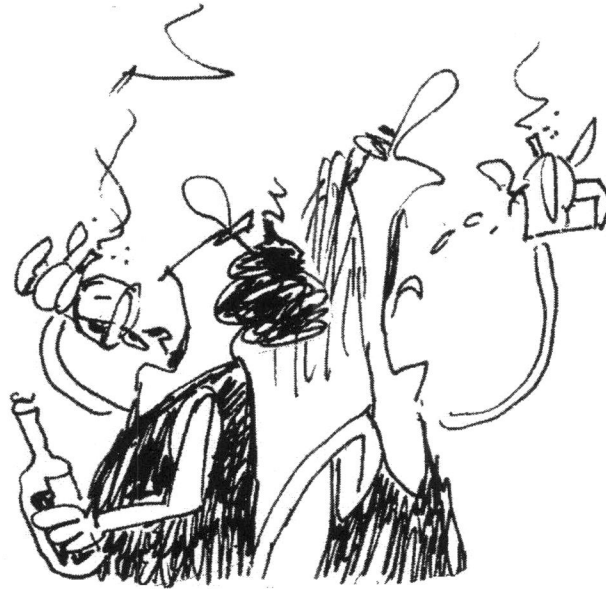

The trick is to limit the overindulgence and spend a little downtime afterward. If you allow the bad eating habits or lack of sleep or whatever your favorite vice may be to build up for more than a day or so, you'll probably end up in a pain crisis, and the strongest medications you've packed won't help.

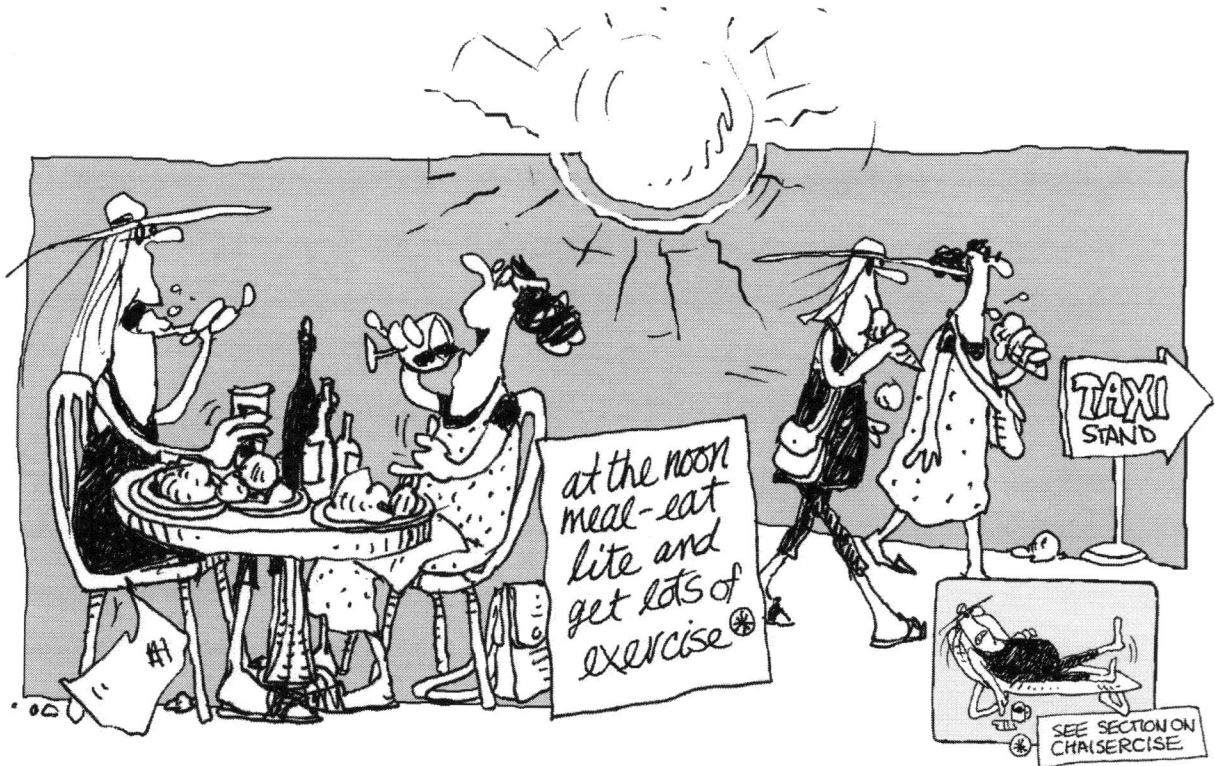

The hospital or doctor's office is not a good place to find yourself at any time, but especially when you're traveling. Either you'll have to take to your bed for an extended and seriously miserable time or you'll end up in the emergency ward begging for help.

The chances of most foreign doctors giving you the heavy medication you need are slim to none. Even if they do give you a powerful injection, you'll have to spend more time unconscious and away from the fun—and the day after you'll feel groggy, irritable and maybe have enough energy to make yourself a coffee. That's two precious days out of your vacation. Was it worth it? Sometimes it is—you be the judge.

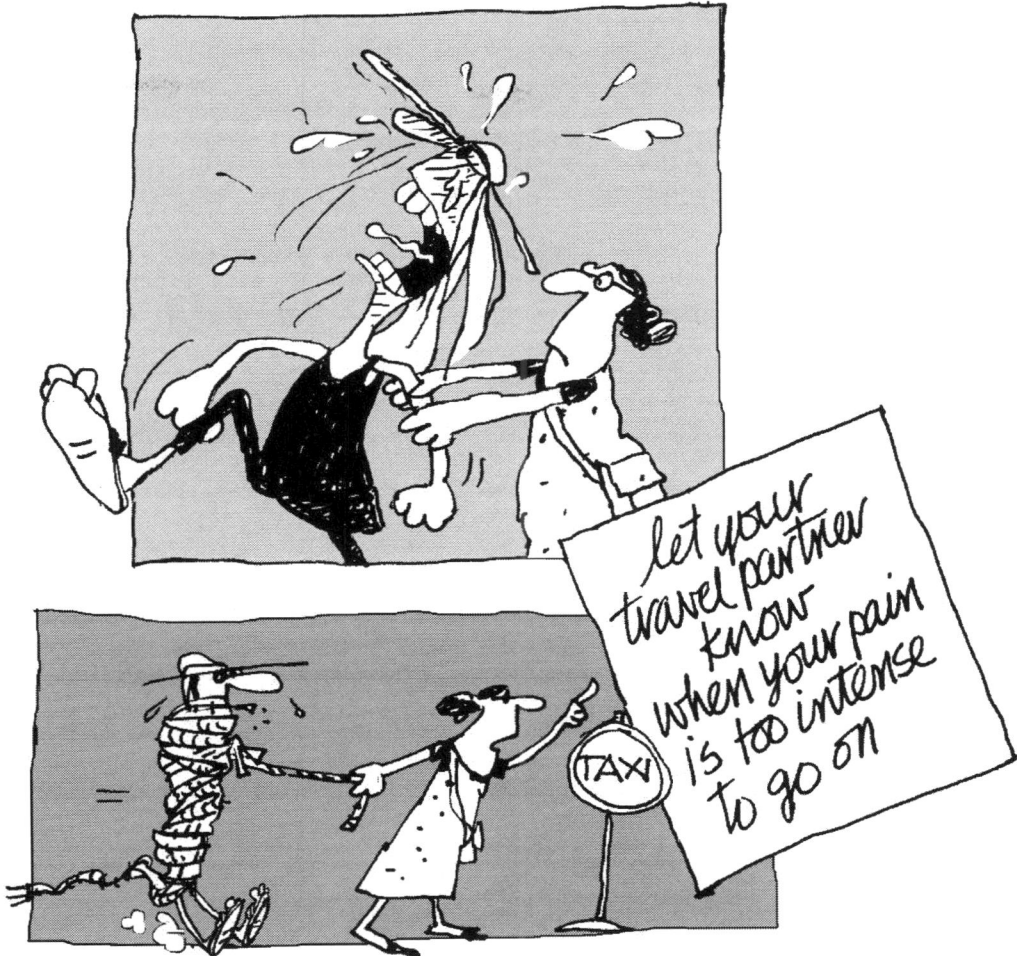

let your travel partner know when your pain is too intense to go on

No one can tell you what you need to do to keep your pain to a minimum; you're the one who knows best from trial and error. The better you feel, the more fun you'll have—that's the ultimate reward.

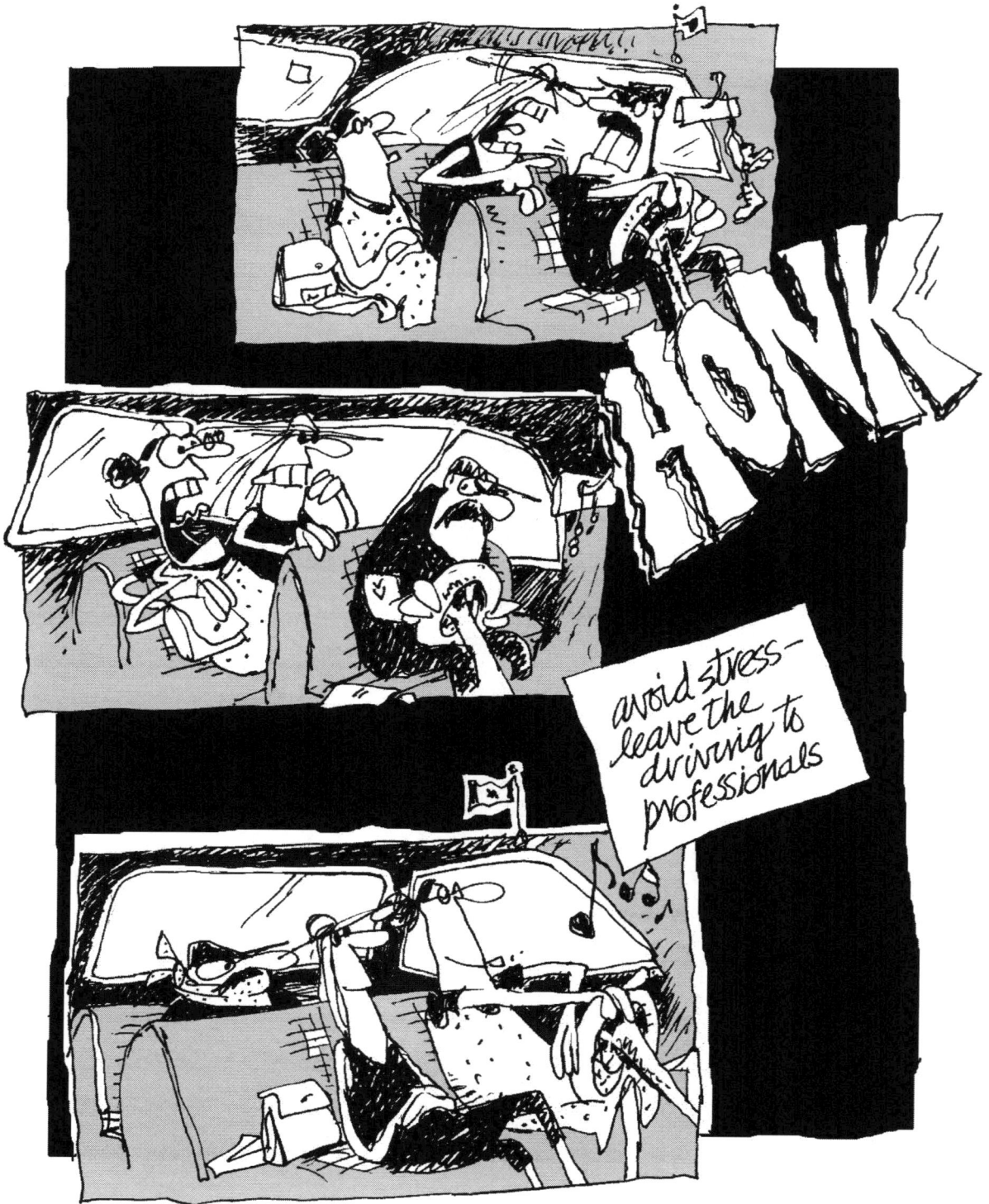

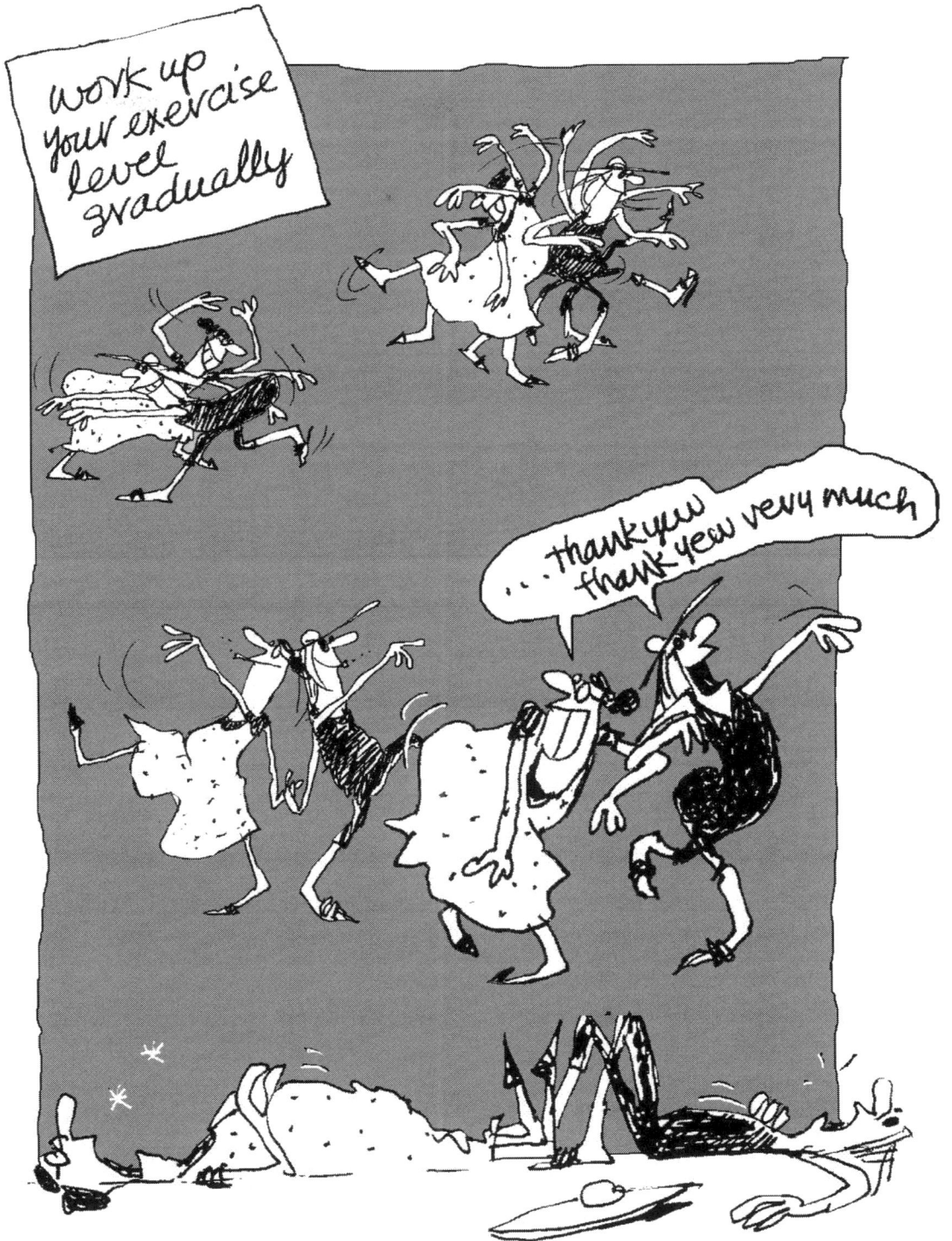

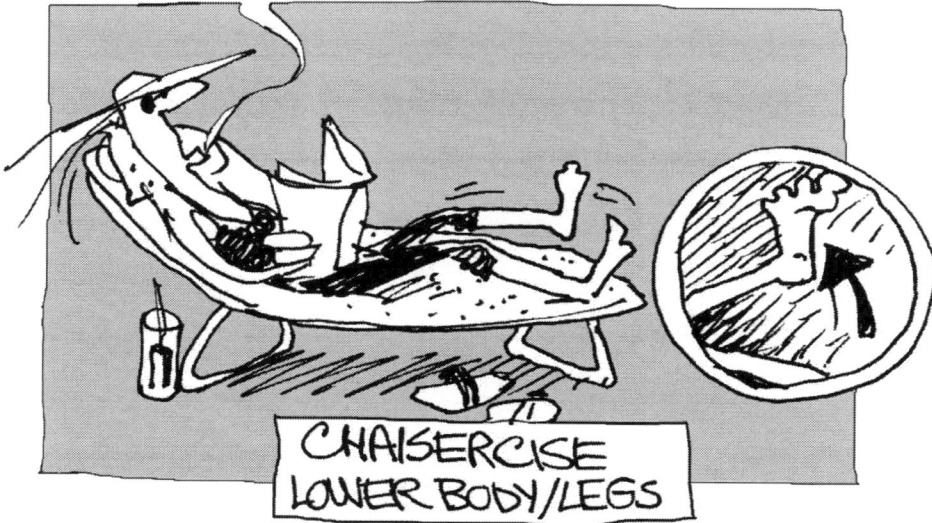

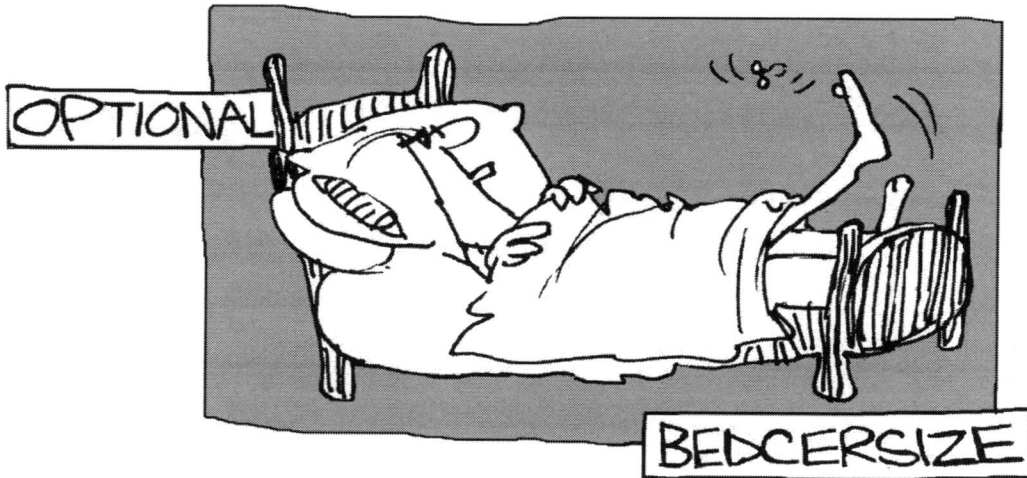

CHAISERCISE
UPPER BODY/ARMS

ADVANCED CHAISERCISE

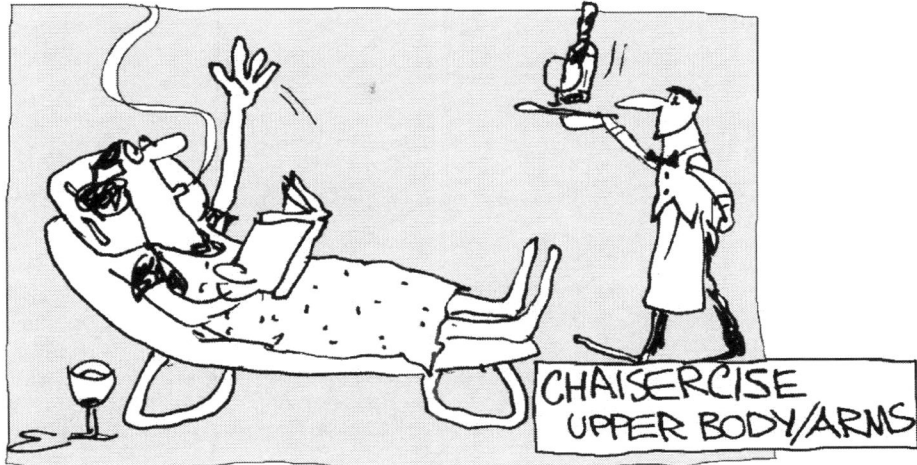

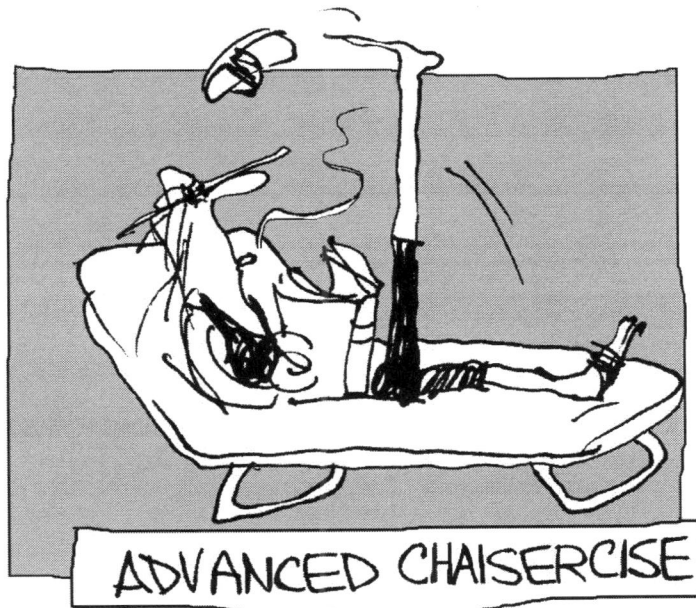

But instead of indulging in too much damaging behavior, try buying yourself a lavish gift or spending the day at a luxurious spa. Hey—we deserve something for putting up with this endless pain! Your body—and probably your Travel Saint— will thank you.

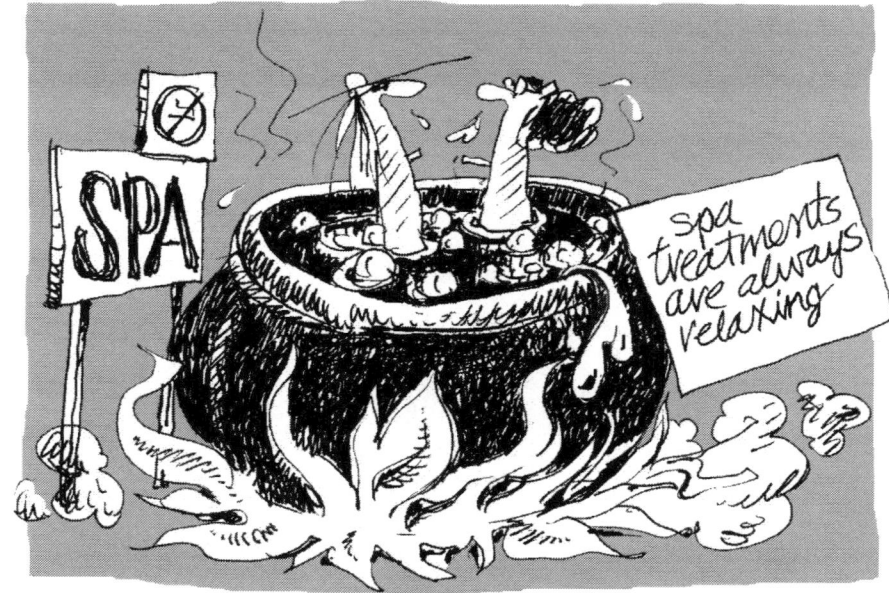

Chapter 12
PAIN & DISCOMFORT

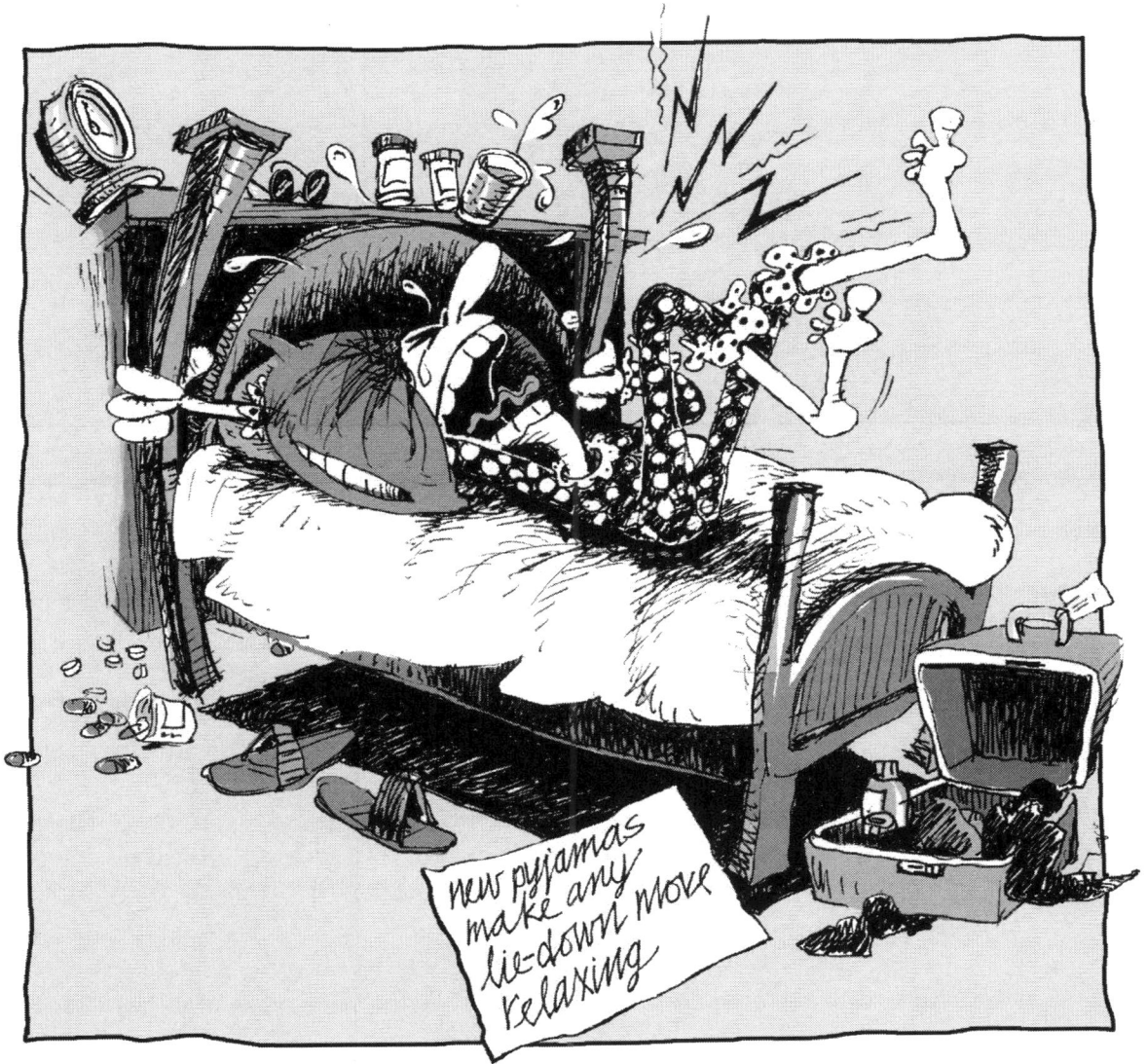

new pyjamas make any lie-down more relaxing

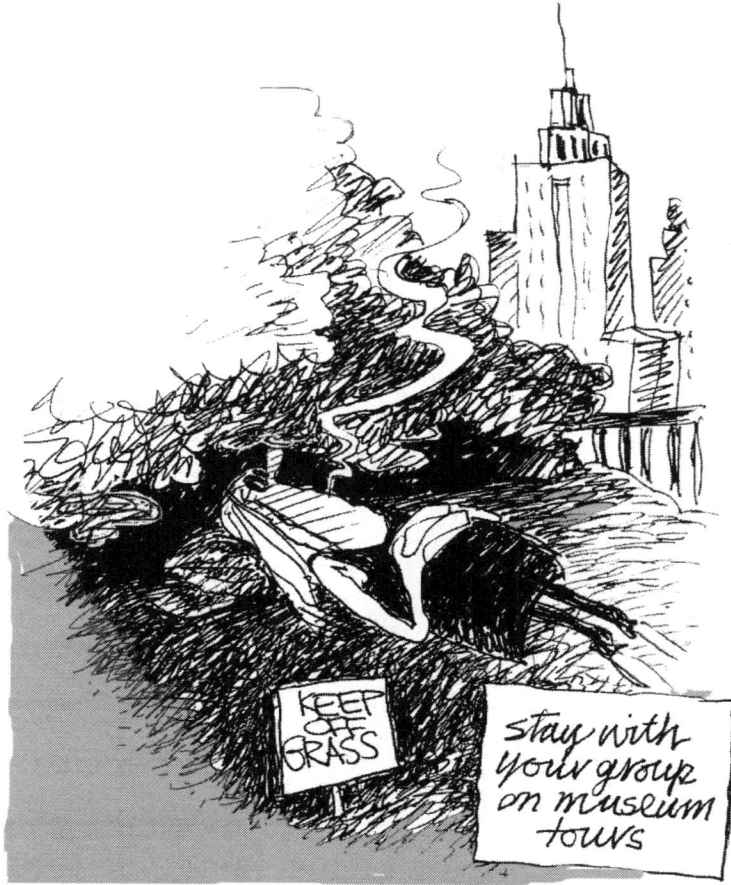

There'll be some. It's a given. If you suffer pain and discomfort at home, you'll suffer from it everywhere else too.

Suffering from chronic pain can be almost like having a split personality. One day you're fine, act normally, can do most of the things everyone else can do. The next day—or often in the middle of something—you're fractured by a pain so intense you have to stop all activity. And until modern science figures it out, you really can't do much about it except take to your bed, gobble pain meds and hope it'll be over soon.

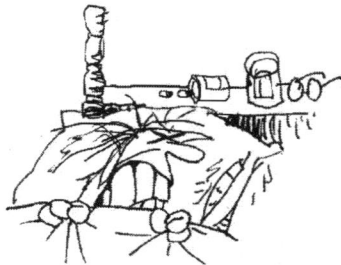

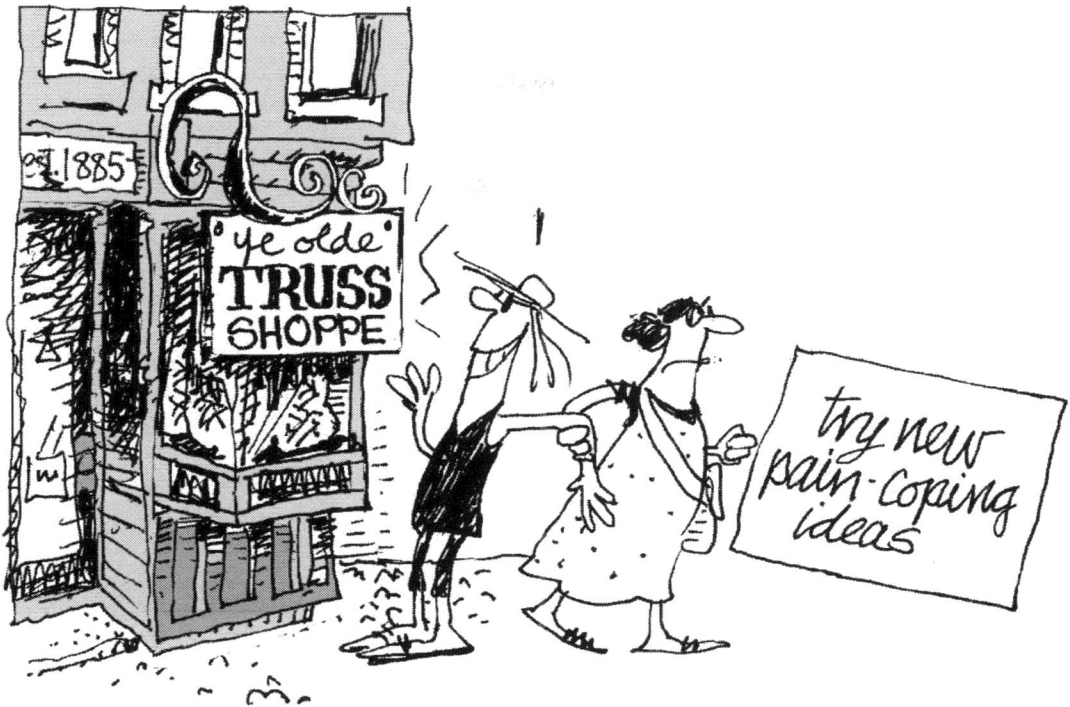

I'm not going to drone on about the various techniques you can use to help with the pain, including hot or cold beanbags, massage, biofeedback, chiropractic, yoga, self-hypnosis or witch-doctory — you know what works and what doesn't, because if you've had chronic pain for any length of time, you've tried almost everything. Whatever works for you, you'll do it — or find it. Unfortunately, no matter what you do or take or have done to you, it will only make the pain slightly more bearable. It won't remove it completely.

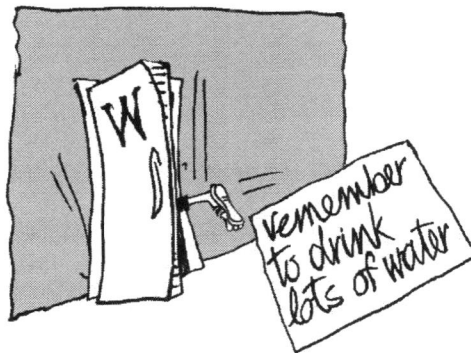

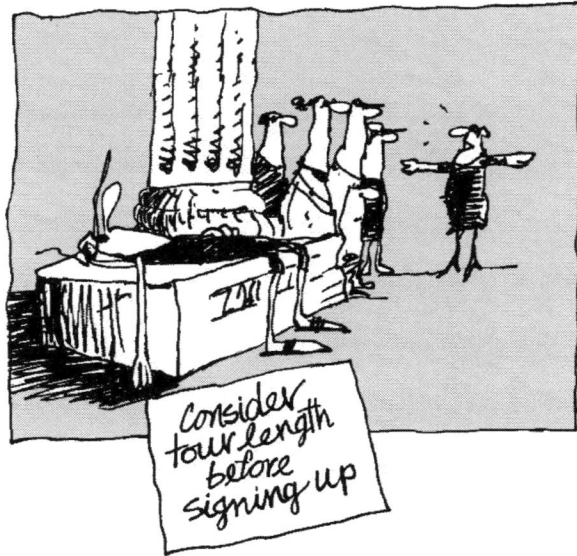

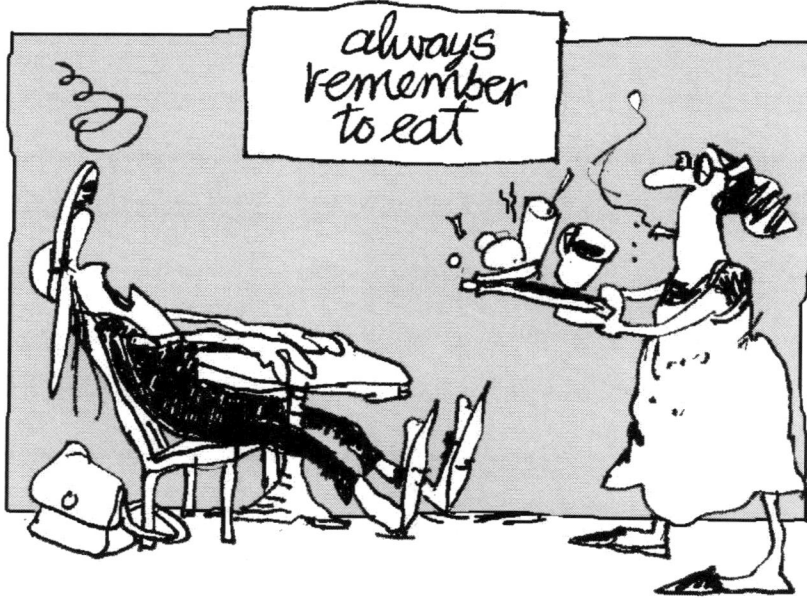

But assuming you'll be down and out occasionally, at other times you'll be up to almost anything.

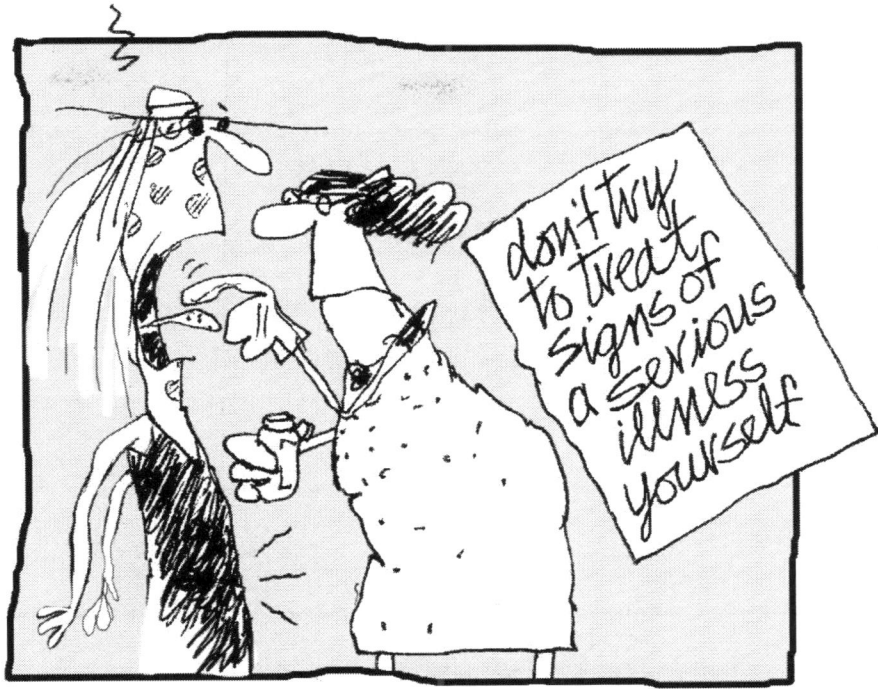

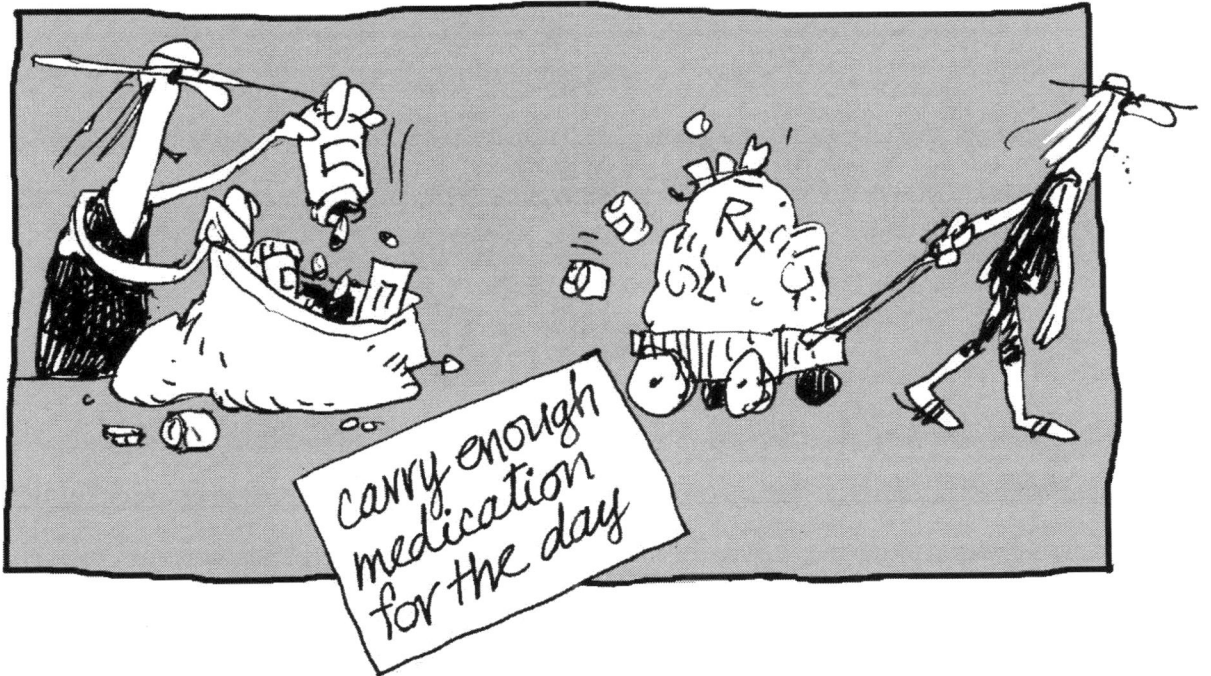

Obviously, some activities, if done to extremes, will bring on a flare-up of your pain.

Don't court agony, but if the only thing you'll suffer from after a night of dancing is slightly sore muscles the next day, it won't kill you. You're on holiday.

On the other hand, if your exertions actually do increase your pain level, stop what you're doing . . . or don't do it so long the next time.

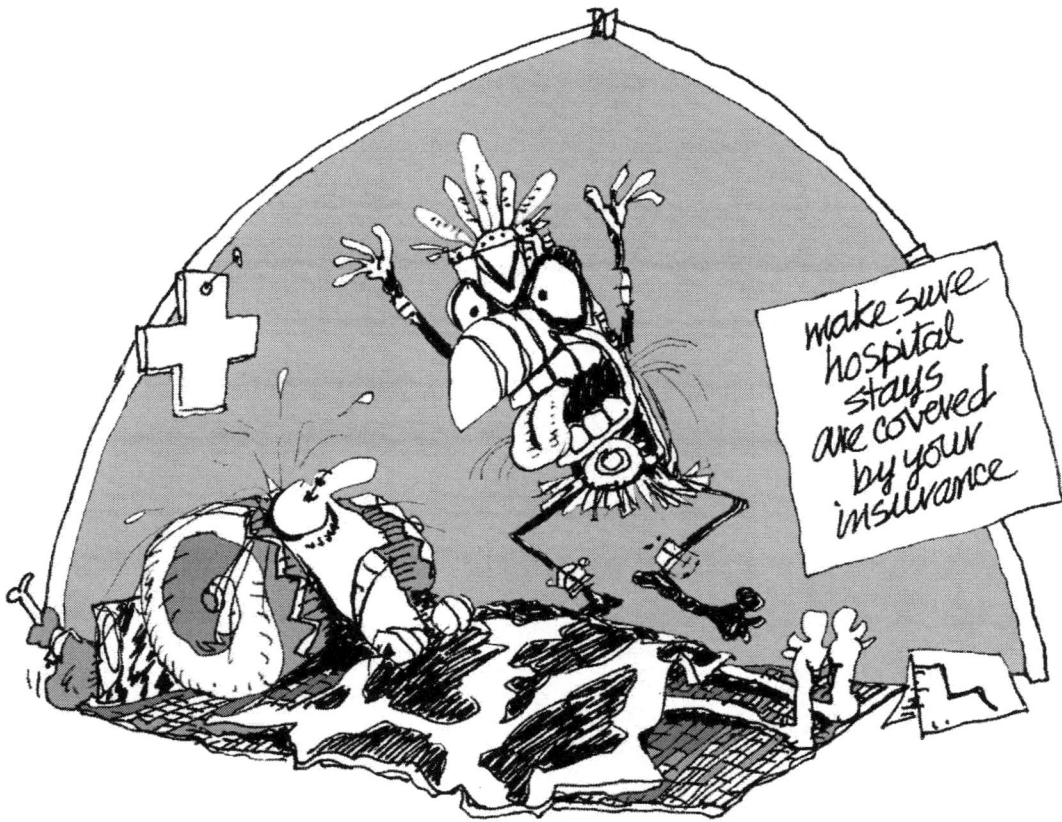

make sure hospital stays are covered by your insurance

Fear of Pain

Chronic pain is usually not constant: it fluctuates from bearable to unbearable and everything in between. But dread of the next painful episode, or fear of pain can be more disabling than the pain itself. And can rob us of far more life than the actual disability.

We may know a lot of the triggers, but we don't always know exactly what will bring on the most severe pain. So even though some days are almost pain-free—or at least bearable—instead of enjoying the day, we start worrying about when the inevitable next attack will come—and where—and we end up sidelining ourselves rather than risk the embarrassment and discomfort of suffering a severe attack far from the security of home.

Perhaps this scientific diagram will help illustrate the point:

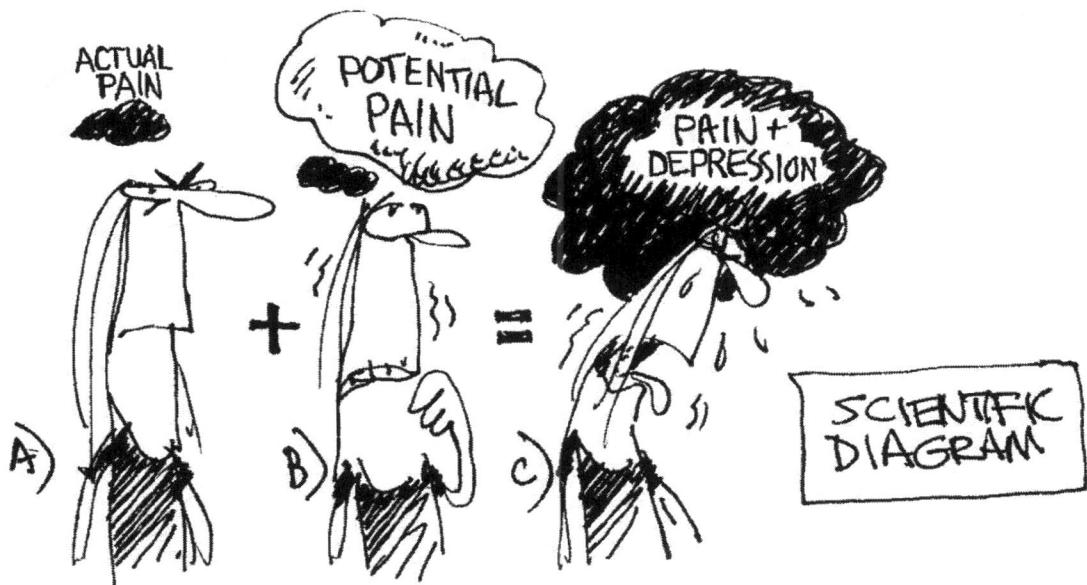

Almost everyone who suffers from chronic pain for any length of time, will give in to this syndrome periodically. But becoming a recluse does not make us better. In fact, it makes the entire thing worse. Not only are we experiencing chronic pain, now we are victims of depression and anxiety as well.

So my motto is "Go for it when you're up to it." That could mean dancing till you drop, or walking up a gentle mountain, or bicycling to a neighboring town or staying up all night to watch a spectacular sunrise. The point is that since you're forced to miss a lot in life, you shouldn't have to miss everything all the time.

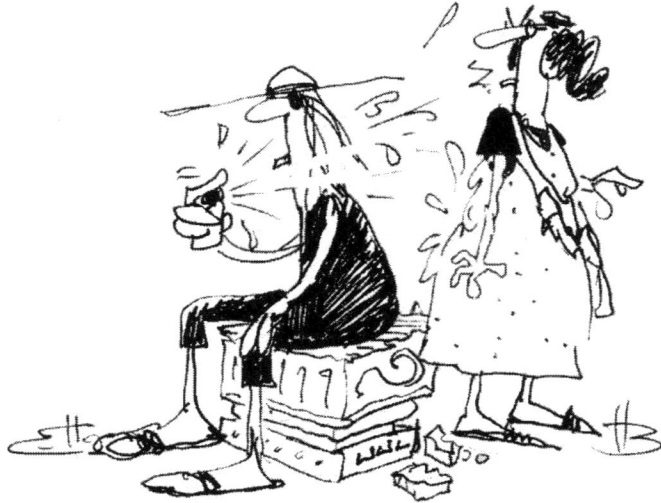

It's of paramount importance to pace yourself. If you're dancing, sit every third dance out or pass on the polka. Drink lots of water. Go outside now and then for some bracing fresh air.

If you're walking or bicycling, take a break once in a while. Even if you were capable of non-stop activity, you'd want to stop and soak in your surroundings.

If you're staying up all night, schedule sleep-in time the next morning (or whenever you finally get to bed).

In other words, if you're doing any fairly strenuous exercise, take a break here and there. In the end, you'll be able to go on far longer, feel much less resultant pain and have a great time doing whatever you're doing.

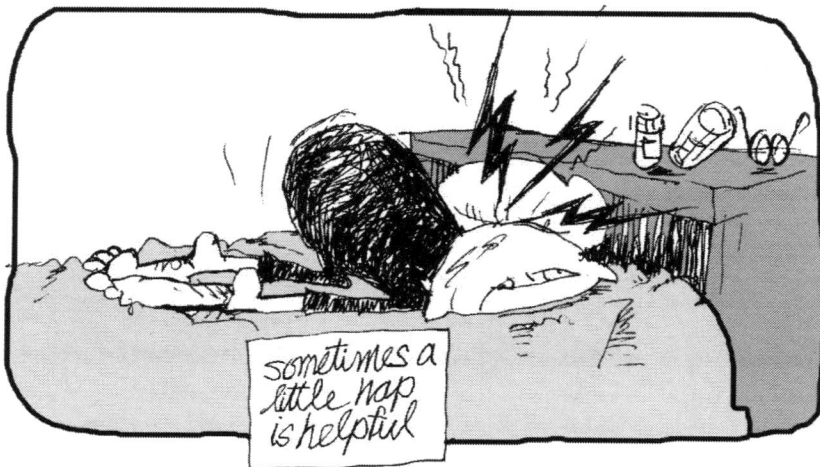

sometimes a little nap is helpful

So yes, there will be times when the pain is almost unendurable—you know this. Give in unapologetically. Your Travel Saint is aware you'll have days like this, and will do whatever possible to make you more comfortable. Your TS can then take off for some sightseeing you weren't that keen on anyway.

If you give in gracefully to the really bad times, you'll suffer far less agony than if you doggedly keep on longer than you should. This is as true at home as it is on vacation.

Remember that pacing is everything, and say YES to as much as you can!

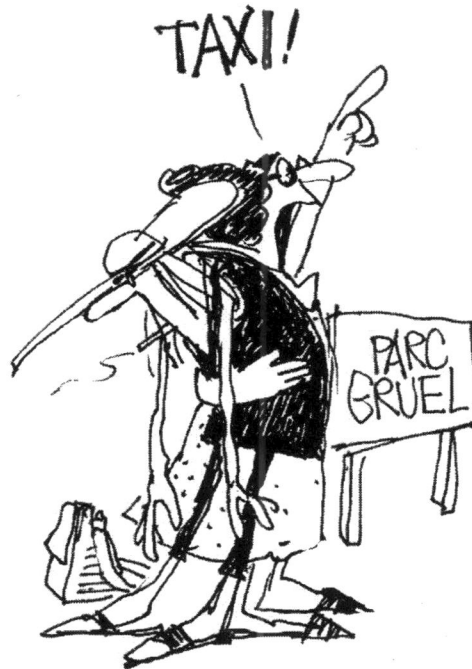

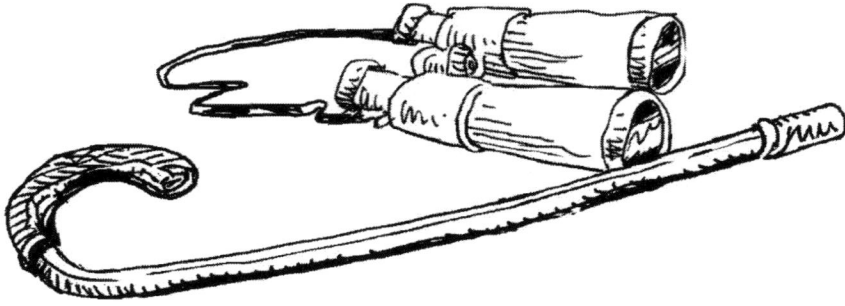

Chapter 13
HOME AGAIN!

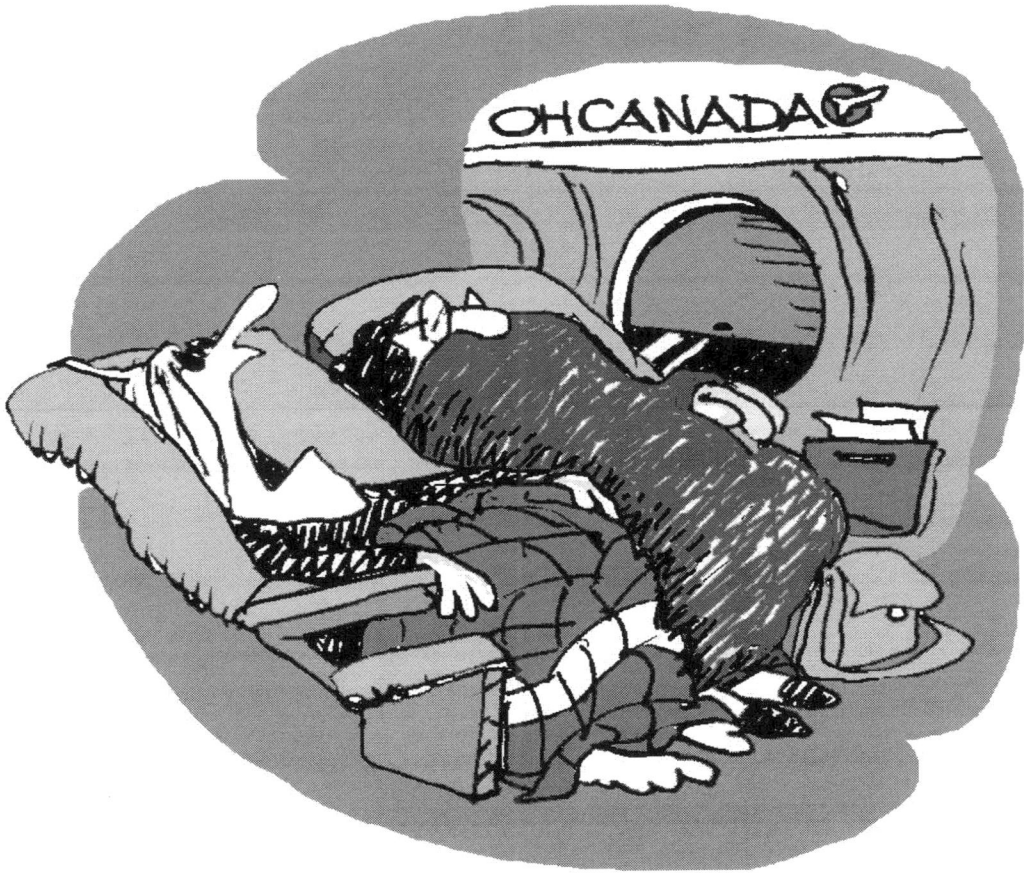

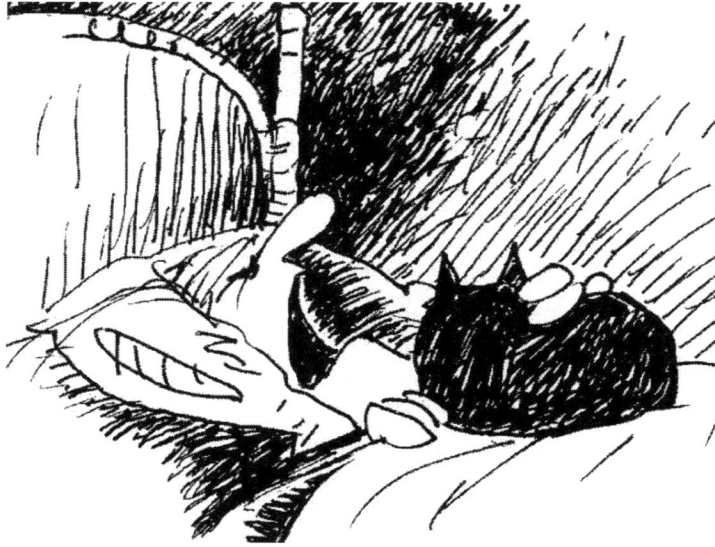

Welcome home! Hide the phone and hit the sack

Finally, after a wonderful, fun-filled, fabulous journey, you're home again! No more maneuvering heavy suitcases through cobble-stoned alleyways, no more tossing and turning on lumpy beds, no more forced joie de vivre when you'd rather be alone. And no more airports, taxis, airplanes, waiting, line-ups—you're home.

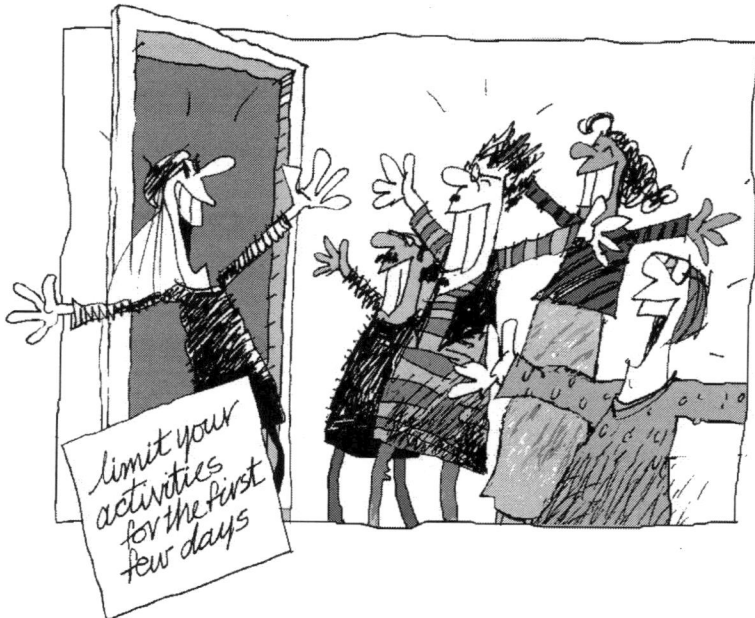

For crying out loud, go to bed. Unpack later. Get as much shut-eye as you can. You'll need it to recover from the almost always arduous trip home. The actual traveling part of travel is difficult and usually painful for anyone with chronic pain, but you made it. Now reward yourself with serious downtime.

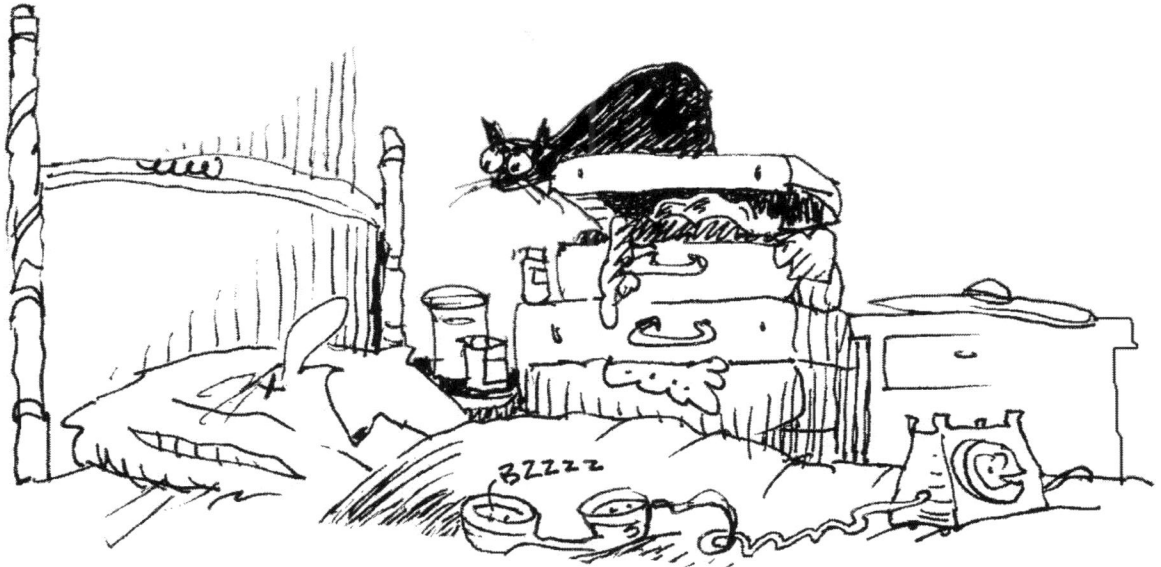

Either tell your co-workers, friends (and family you don't live with) that you'll be in touch a few days after your return, or let everyone know that you'll be home two days later than your actual arrival. It's very important that you get over jet lag in a natural way, adjust your daily rhythms back to your real-life schedule and readjust to climate, barometric pressures and anything else that's radically different at home than where you've been.

And let's face it, traveling requires a level of sociability that you might not choose in your normal life. You'll probably be worn out. Turn off the phone and climb into the sack.

If you live alone, arrange with a good friend who understands your need for recuperative time to stock your fridge and cupboard with a few essentials so you don't have to run out to the store immediately. And if you put clean sheets on your bed, clean PJs under the pillow and an extra toothbrush in the bathroom before you left, you're ready to fall into bed when you get back. You won't need to unpack anything except your meds—and that's easy because they're in your carry-on.

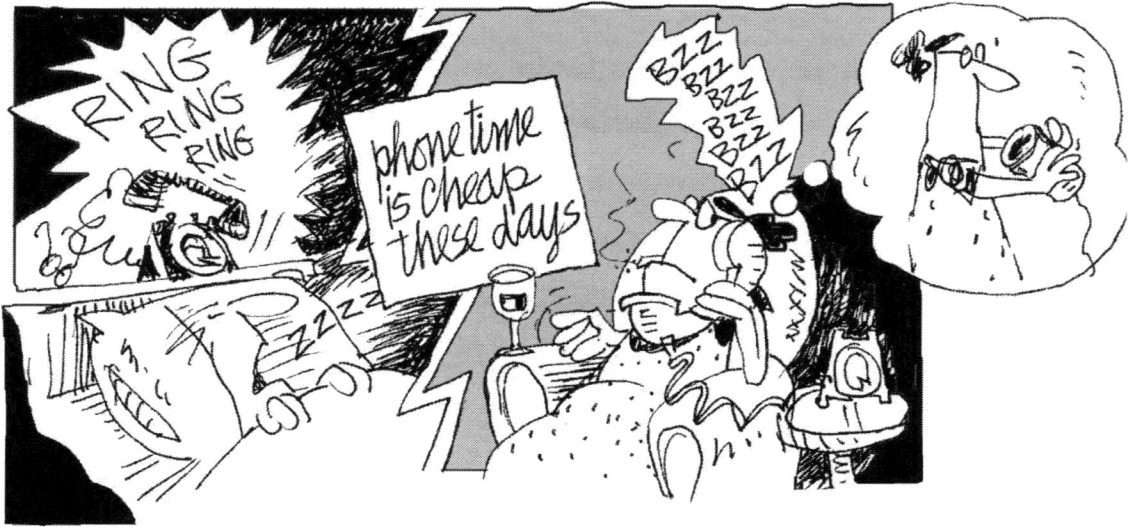

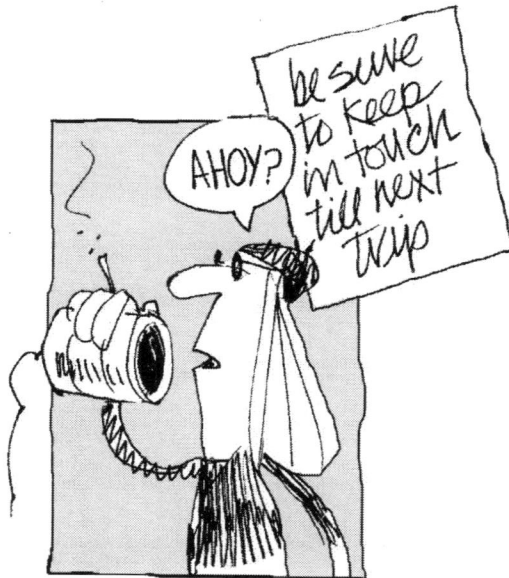

Once you've recuperated, you're rested, happy to be home and anxious to see people. Still, it's a good idea not to cram too much into the first few days. You've probably been used to a slightly more active life while away and you may have built up a tolerance for doing things, going places and seeing people that you didn't have previously. But in case this new ability to go on and on is not sustainable long term but was a marathon you managed to do while away, test the waters before committing to too much too soon. You may prefer your old pace—or you may discover previously untold reserves of energy.

140

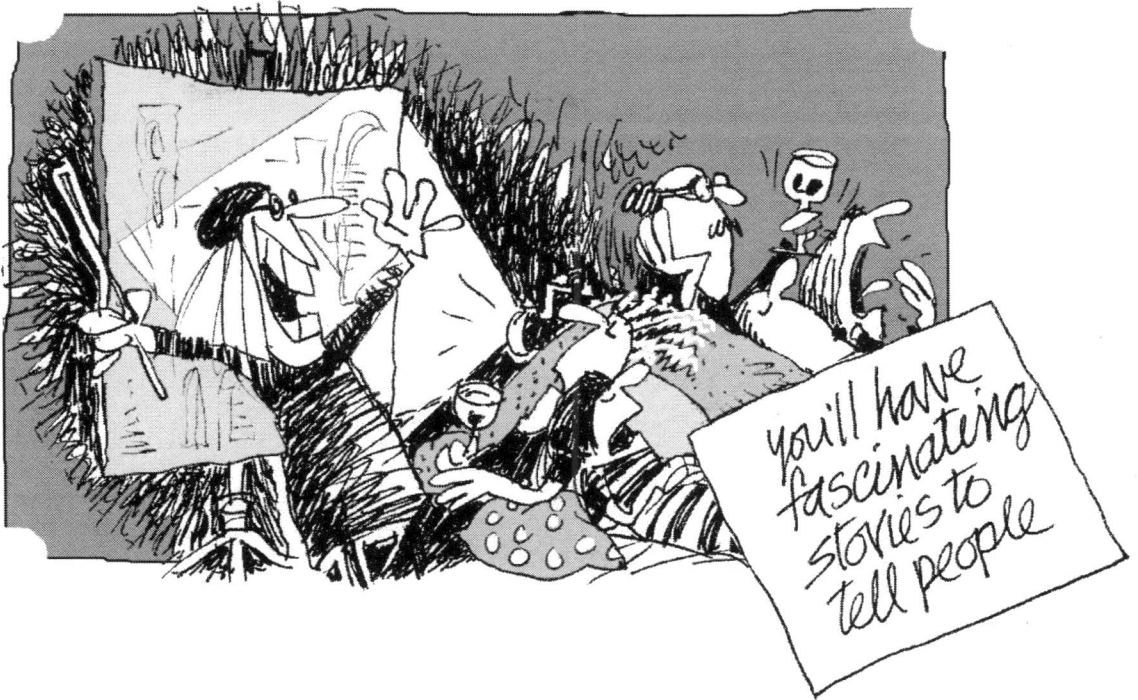

you'll have fascinating stories to tell people

It's a wonderful feeling to plan a holiday, go somewhere different, see new people, places and things. And it's an especially wonderful feeling of accomplishment that you did all that while suffering from chronic pain. Be proud of yourself, enjoy telling the stories and showing the pictures.

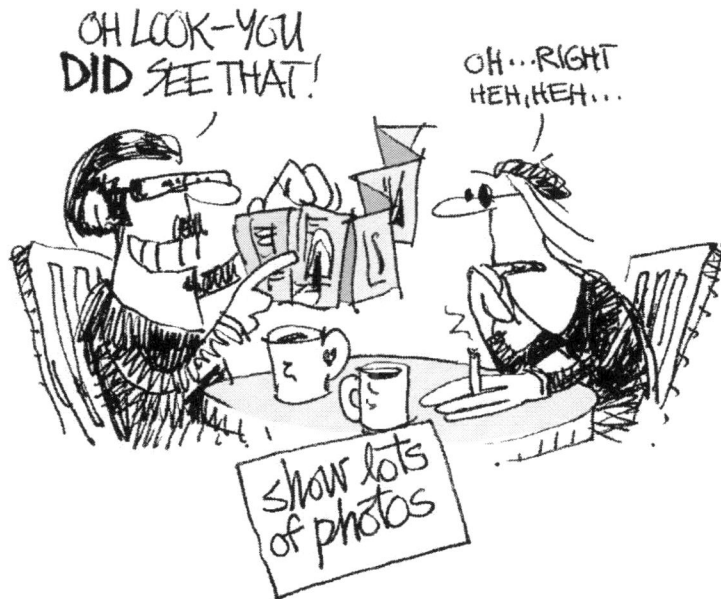

OH LOOK—YOU DID SEE THAT!

OH…RIGHT HEH, HEH…

show lots of photos

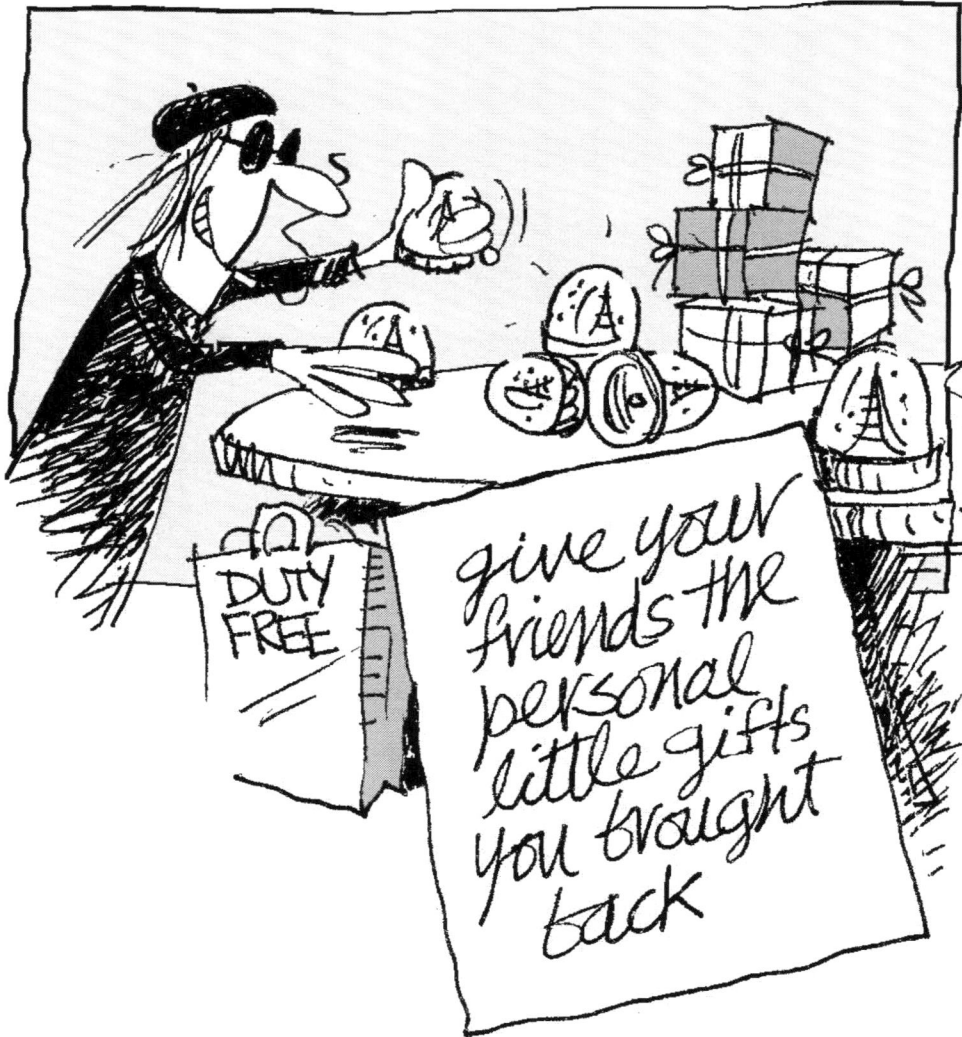

give your friends the personal little gifts you brought back

You may not feel like it right away, but it won't be long before you're planning another fabulous journey to a brand new destination. Congratulations and welcome home!

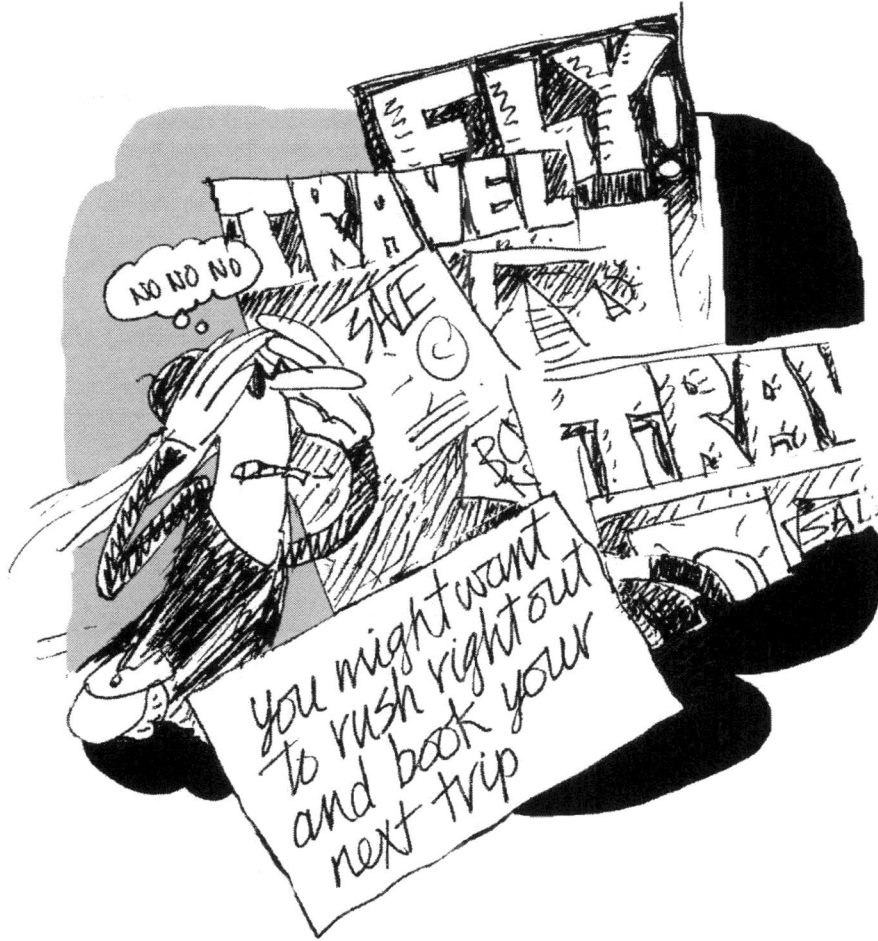

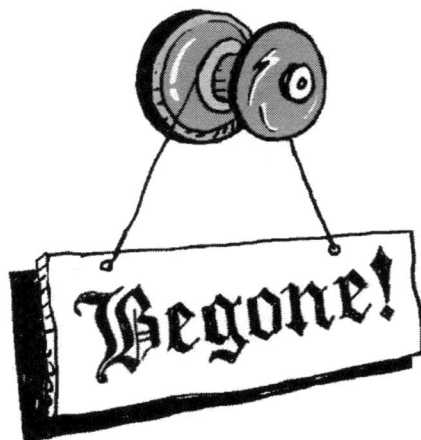

Chapter 14
THE WISH LIST

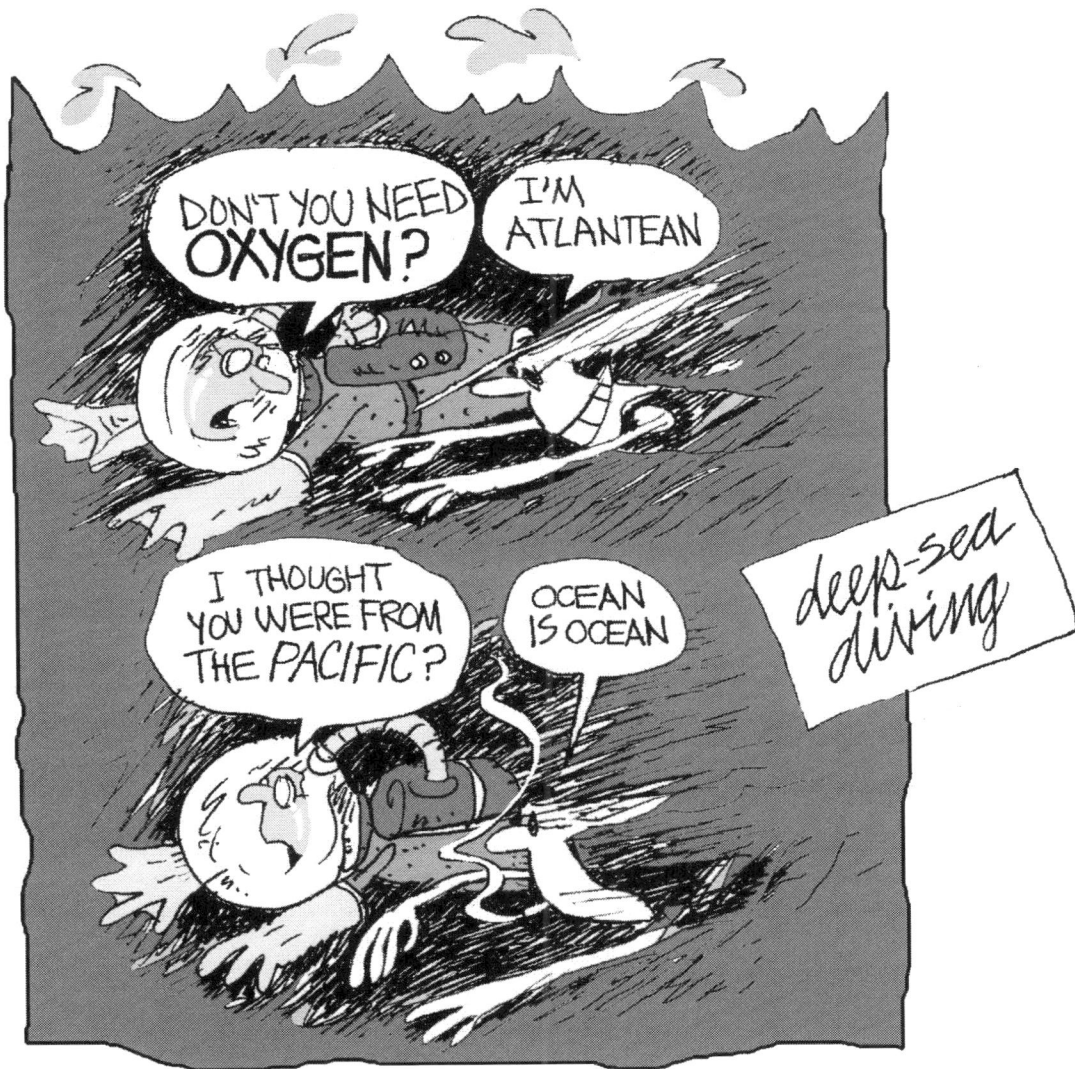

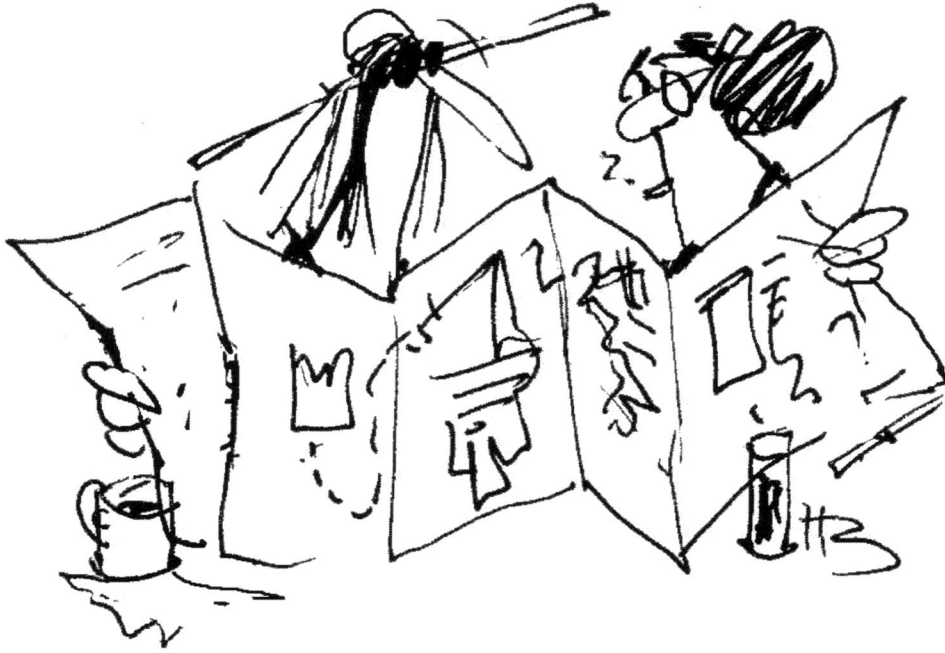

On the other hand…Maybe anything's possible

When I first started this book, I thought if I could share what I've learned over the decades, maybe I could help other people who suffer from chronic pain see that it's possible to travel, possible to do lots of things despite the almost constant pain. And as a cartoonist, I saw the lighter side of the depressing reality—because there's always a funny side, if you look for it.

But an unexpected thing happened. As I wrote and drew and thought about all the ways we could get around the problems of travel, I started to feel like it was not only possible for me to do regular trips, but maybe I could even do more difficult things—like travel to really hot countries. Do an Amazon boat trip. Go to space sometime in the future. Maybe manage destinations I'd previously thought were impossible given my daily pain.

I've always wanted, more than anywhere on earth, to go to Egypt. Actually, ancient Egypt, but as time travel seems out of the question so far, I'd be happy with modern-day Egypt as long as I spend most of my time exploring antiquities.

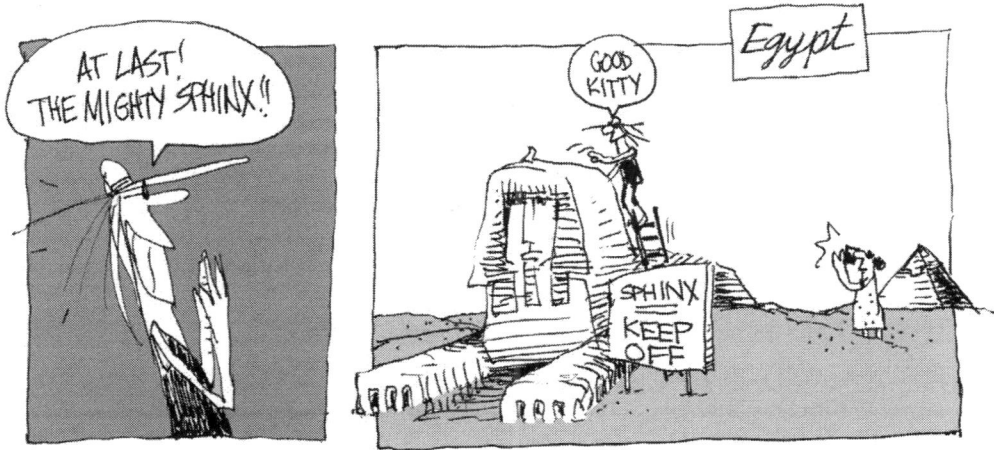

Unfortunately—aside from pesky social upheaval, wars and whatnot—Egypt is in the desert. Hot. Horrendously hot. And I don't do hot well. But the last time I was in southern Spain, it was close to 100°F, and the Travel Saint and I managed somehow. How much worse could Egypt be?

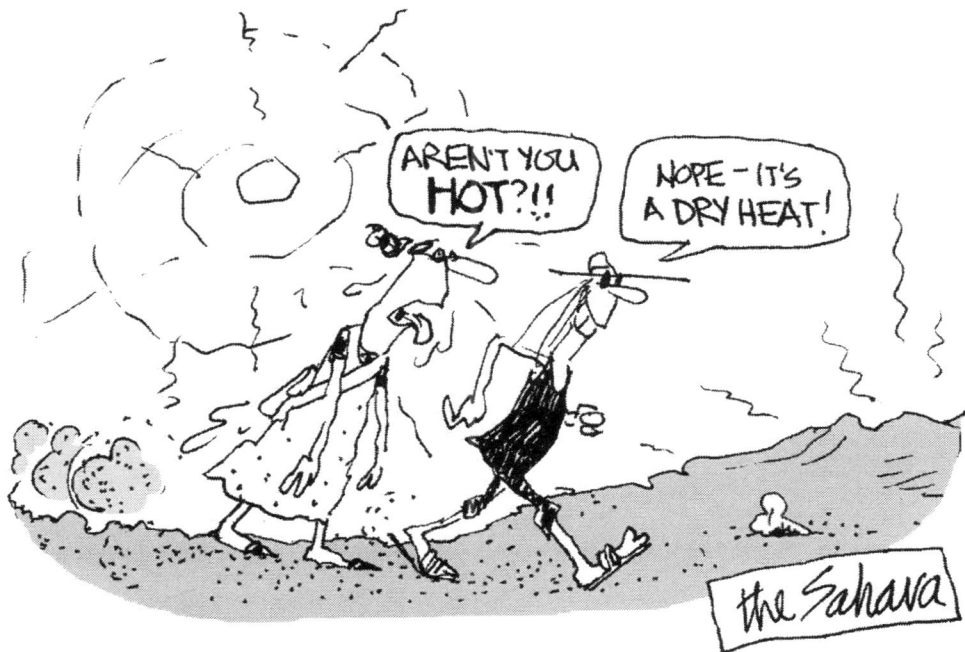

Conversely, I'd love to spend a few nights in an ice hotel, one of those fabulous palaces made entirely from ice: beds, floors, tables, chairs, even cocktails served in an ice glass. With candlelight dancing off the ice facets, it must be like hanging out in a diamond!

I live in Canada (on the West Coast), and Quebec City in the Province of Quebec boasts Canada's first ice hotel, a tourist "hot spot." I love Quebec, but a hotel made entirely of ice has to be freezing, no? Even with fireplaces everywhere, overnight guests wear long underwear and sleep in mummy bags although the hotel also has heated rooms for the not-so-brave. Yes, I hate cold almost as much as heat, and my daily headaches increase significantly in extreme temperatures and climatic changes, but . . . my head's going to ache anyway no matter where I am . . . at least I'd wake up in a crystal palace!

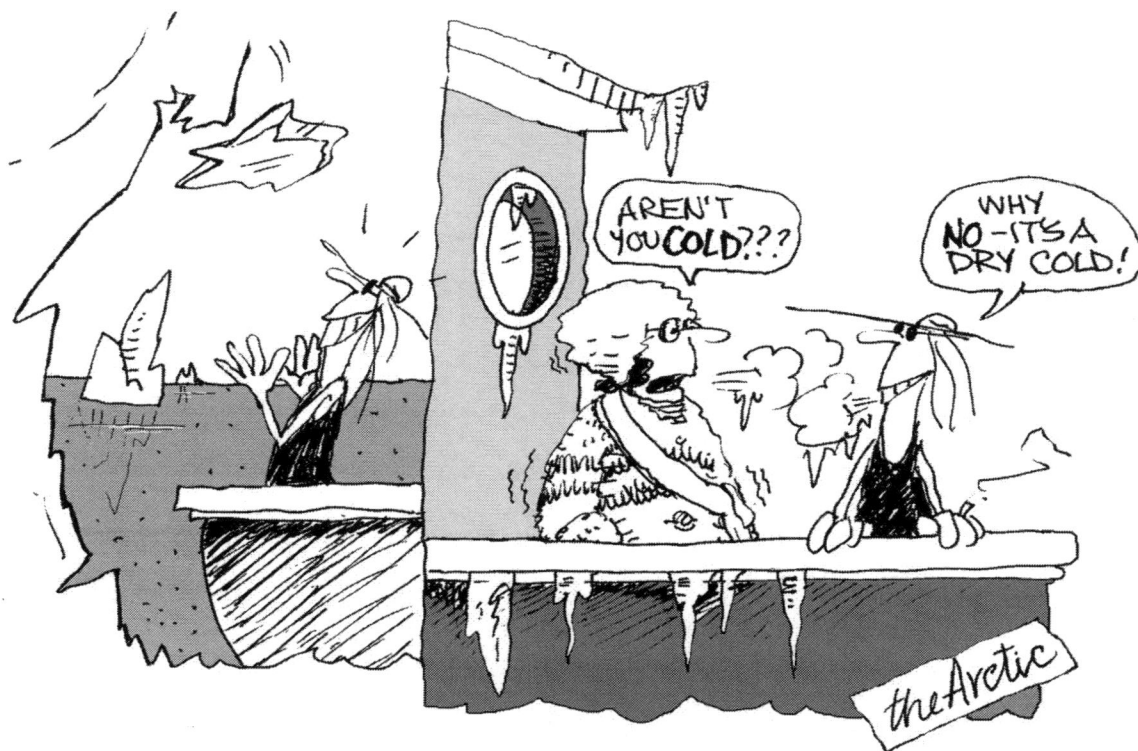

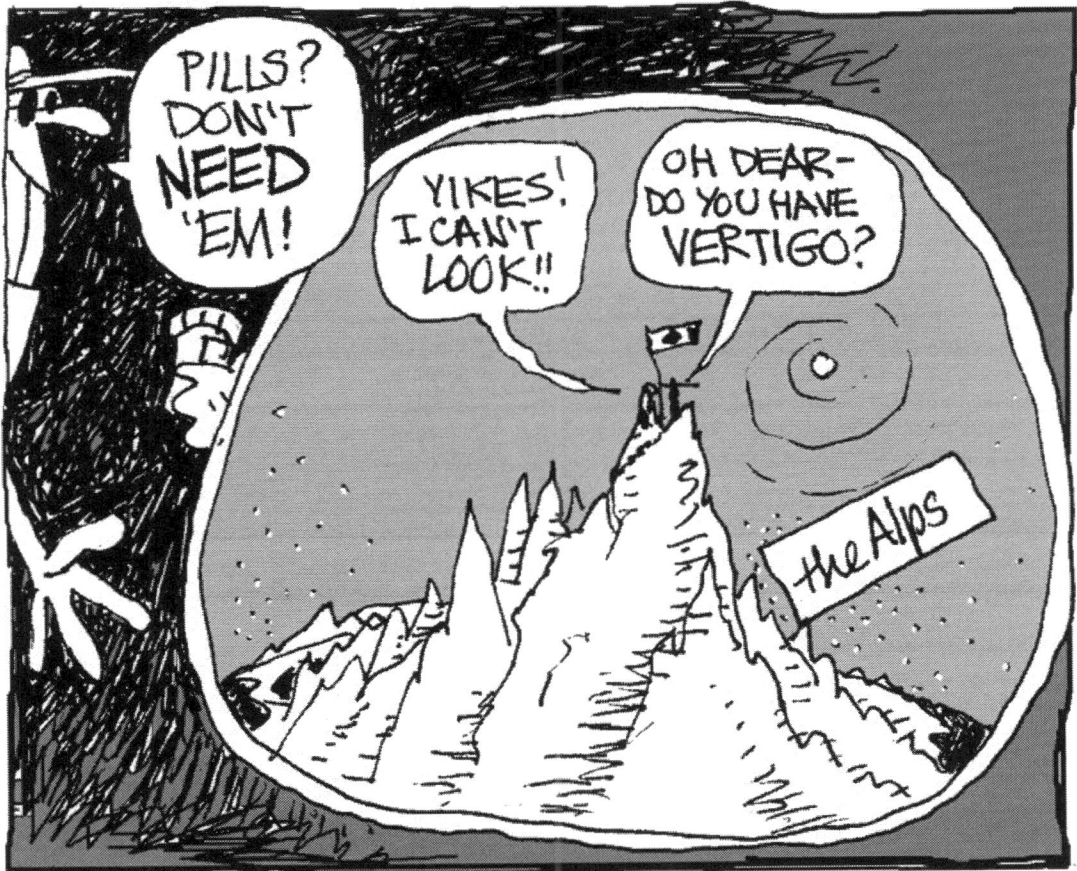

I've been across Canada and the US a number of times and to temperate places like Alaska (in summer), Britain, France, and Switzerland as well as warmer spots like Italy, Spain, Greece, Mexico, Jamaica, the Bahamas, Santa Fe and various other hot places, although I do tend to travel in the off season when it's cooler. I've spent time in New Orleans and absolutely loved it, though my pain was pretty severe. I'd really like to go back to Louisiana, then on to Georgia and spend time in the deep South. But there's that heat thing again—even worse than desert heat, in a way: the humidity, the humidity! Ah lord, the humidity! (Gasp!)

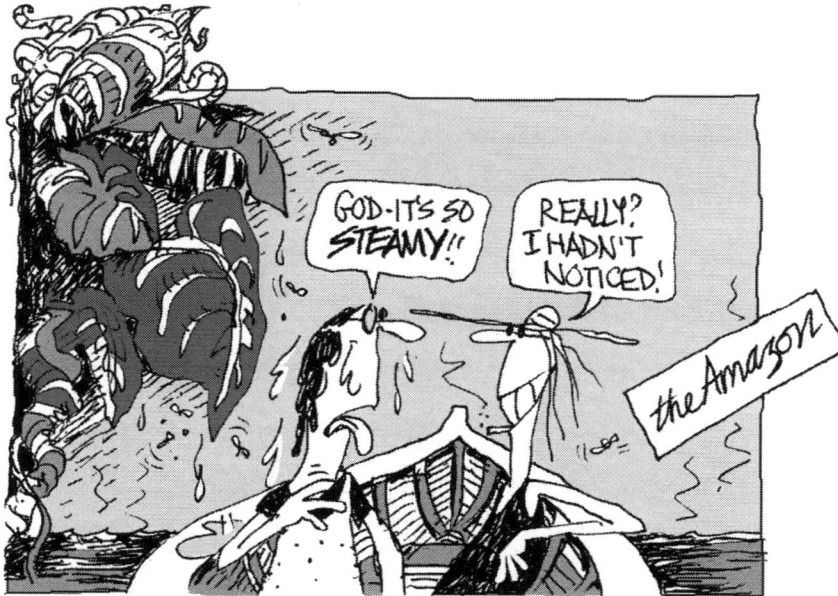

So OK, maybe the Amazon would be pushing it. Maybe an Arctic trek across the glaciers, watching icebergs calve in the fjords, is not a great idea. Perhaps it's too far to Peru. But just maybe, if I save up my travel bucks for a long time and go pretty much first class, I can guarantee a lot of air conditioning and central heating, possibly climate-controlled limos. Or perhaps I could wear a designer hazmat suit. I don't know. But I'm keeping my options open and my fingers crossed.

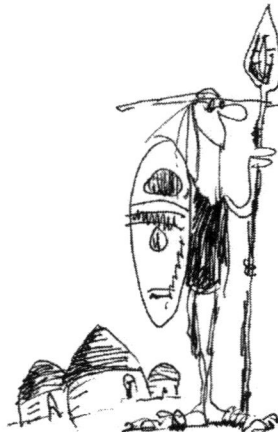

In the meantime, I have so many places yet to explore where I could be comfortable.

I'll go to them first.

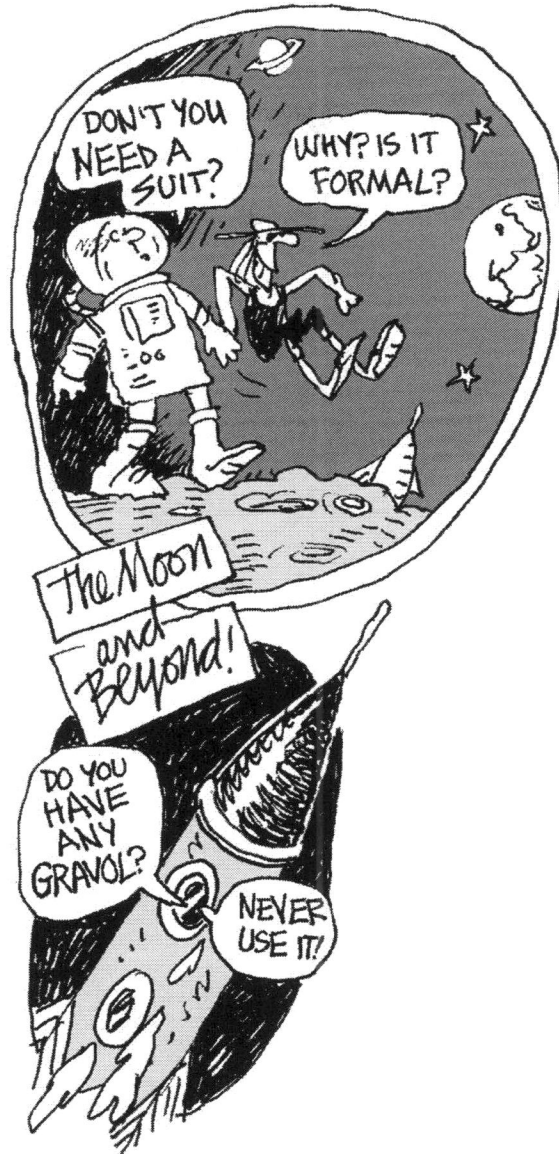

So pack up your meds and your back boards and your folding canes, and I'll see you there!

"Bon voyage" to you and me—intrepid travelers who see as much of the world as we can when we can . . . if chronic pain forces us to live a half-life, at least we'll live our half to the fullest. And that's doing a lot more living than many people who've never had a serious pain in their lives.

Happy Trails!

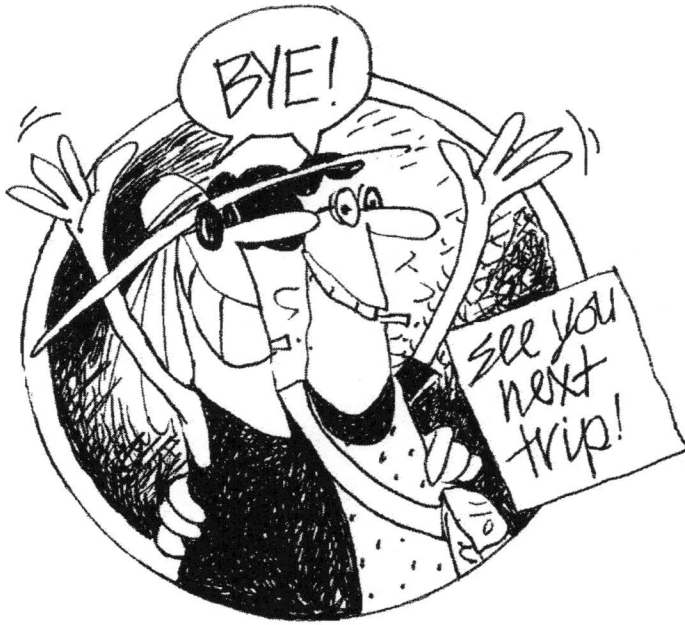

APPENDIX
10 WAYS TO COPE WITH CHRONIC PAIN

These suggestions are meant more for living a life than strictly for travel. But if we can't figure out some way to deal with the pain, it's likely we're not going anywhere—other than bed or the hospital.

I am not a doctor or medical person of any kind. I am someone who's suffered from chronic pain all my adult life and a significant part of my childhood. I've seen and been seen by many, many health professionals in a sometimes desperate attempt to have my pain diagnosed and more importantly, cured. Unfortunately, although the diagnosis was fairly straightforward, there is no real cure for my specific malady.

Nevertheless, over the years, I've come across strategies, medical procedures, drugs and various other coping mechanisms—some actually help. None entirely rid me of pain. Because chronic pain can affect every aspect of our lives, it's important that the people you're closest to understand your affliction. In the hopes that my experience will be of use to some of you, here are my suggestions for dealing with chronic pain.

1. Seek Medical Advice

Be very honest about your pain. Your doctor may recommend various tests to find the underlying problem. He or she will tell you if there are any medical procedures that will help.

2. Confide

Find a trusted friend, therapist or support group. It's helpful to have someone you can talk to about the pain. It's useful to know that others are suffering the same way you are and you may find new ways of coping that work for others in similar situations.

3. Research

The Internet is full of information on your particular pain. Refine your search; for example, type into your search engine, "coping with Bursitis" or "non-medical tips for chronic bursitis pain". The more specific your search, the more targeted information you'll find.

4. Homeopathic & Alternative Medicine

Many types of chronic pain are helped by chiropractic, acupuncture, massage, physical therapy, bio-feedback, etc. Be open to trying trusted, alternative coping methods for your pain.

5. Pharmaceuticals

If the pain is so severe that it limits your lifestyle significantly, ask your doctor to prescribe pain medication. Handled carefully, narcotics and other pain medication can give you back your life.

6. Employment Difficulty

Chronic pain often makes it impossible to hold a 9-to-5 job. Consider employment options like job-sharing, freelancing or discussing less rigid hours with your employer.

7. Financial Assistance

If your pain is so great and so frequent that it affects your ability to make a living, explore your government's social assistance programs.

8. Relationships

Some pain medications affect the libido, some are mood-altering, and chronic pain itself sometimes alters our ability to interact with others. If you notice difficulties in any area of your relationships, talk to people frankly about your condition. When friends and loved ones know why you sometimes have difficulty responding normally, they will understand it's not personal and will give you time to recover until you're yourself again.

9. Depression

Depression is a side effect of chronic pain. Talking about it helps. But if the depression becomes as much a problem as the pain itself, seek therapy and/or ask your doctor to prescribe pharmaceutical relief.

10. Anger

It's natural to feel angry when it seems there's just no cure for your pain and you'll have to endure it either forever or until they find a cure. The tension of anger can significantly intensify the pain. When the anger threatens to engulf you, try to find a trusted friend who can talk you through it. If that's not possible, watch a very funny comedy. Laughter really is the best medicine.

(And of course, count your blessings. Sometimes it helps put our pain in perspective when we remember there are always people living with much worse conditions.)

ABOUT THE AUTHOR

wendy brown is the recipient of over fourteen provincial, national and international newspaper editorial cartooning awards. She writes, paints and lives with her cat, Edward, in a small town on the Pacific coast in British Columbia, Canada. Originally from Toronto, where she studied fine art at OCAD, brown worked as an art director, illustrator and cartoonist in advertising and publishing until she moved to BC with her son in the 1990s.

brown is currently at work on a collection of short stories, a comic novel and a sequel to OWww! She continues to groan her way around the world whenever she feels the need to leave town.

www.wendybrown.ca
https://www.facebook.com/OWww-625302254159904/
http://claremark.ca/nobots/wendybrown/

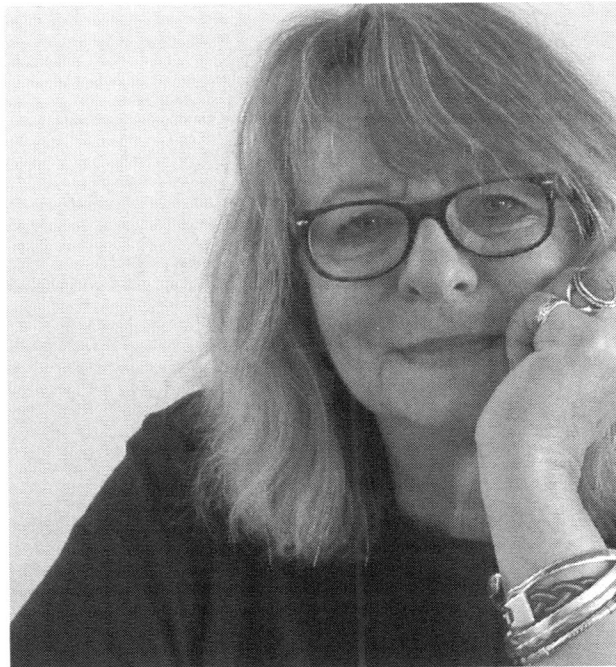

Made in the USA
Columbia, SC
06 October 2017